A NURSE'S
▶ ▶ ▶ STEP ▶ BY ▶ STEP ▶ ▶ ▶
GUIDE TO

TRANSITIONING TO AN ACADEMIC ROLE

Strategies to Jumpstart Your Career
in Education and Research

MERCY NGOSA MUMBA, PhD, RN, CMSRN, FAAN

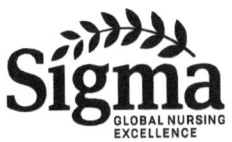

Copyright © 2022 by Sigma Theta Tau International Honor Society of Nursing

All rights reserved. This book is protected by copyright. No part of it may be reproduced, stored in a retrieval system, or transmitted in any form or by any means, electronic, mechanical, photocopying, recording, or otherwise, without written permission from the publisher. Any trademarks, service marks, design rights, or similar rights that are mentioned, used, or cited in this book are the property of their respective owners. Their use here does not imply that you may use them for a similar or any other purpose.

This book is not intended to be a substitute for the medical advice of a licensed medical professional. The author and publisher have made every effort to ensure the accuracy of the information contained within at the time of its publication and shall have no liability or responsibility to any person or entity regarding any loss or damage incurred, or alleged to have incurred, directly or indirectly, by the information contained in this book. The author and publisher make no warranties, express or implied, with respect to its content, and no warranties may be created or extended by sales representatives or written sales materials. The author and publisher have no responsibility for the consistency or accuracy of URLs and content of third-party websites referenced in this book.

Sigma Theta Tau International Honor Society of Nursing (Sigma) is a nonprofit organization whose mission is developing nurse leaders anywhere to improve healthcare everywhere. Founded in 1922, Sigma has more than 135,000 active members in over 100 countries and territories. Members include practicing nurses, instructors, researchers, policymakers, entrepreneurs, and others. Sigma's more than 540 chapters are located at more than 700 institutions of higher education throughout Armenia, Australia, Botswana, Brazil, Canada, Colombia, Croatia, England, Eswatini, Ghana, Hong Kong, Ireland, Israel, Italy, Jamaica, Japan, Jordan, Kenya, Lebanon, Malawi, Mexico, the Netherlands, Nigeria, Pakistan, Philippines, Portugal, Puerto Rico, Scotland, Singapore, South Africa, South Korea, Sweden, Taiwan, Tanzania, Thailand, the United States, and Wales. Learn more at www.sigmanursing.org.

Sigma Theta Tau International
550 West North Street
Indianapolis, IN, USA 46202

To request a review copy for course adoption, order additional books, buy in bulk, or purchase for corporate use, contact Sigma Marketplace at 888.654.4964 (US/Canada toll-free), +1.317.687.2256 (International), or solutions@sigmamarketplace.org.

To request author information, or for speaker or other media requests, contact Sigma Marketing at 888.634.7575 (US/Canada toll-free) or +1.317.634.8171 (International).

ISBN: 9781646480296
EPUB ISBN: 9781646480319
PDF ISBN: 9781646480326

Library of Congress Control Number: 2022009480

First Printing, 2022

Publisher: Dustin Sullivan
Acquisitions Editor: Emily Hatch
Development Editor: Meaghan O'Keeffe
Cover Designer: Rebecca Batchelor
Interior Design/Page Layout: Rebecca Batchelor
Indexer: Larry Sweazy

Managing Editor: Carla Hall
Publications Specialist: Todd Lothery
Project Editor: Meaghan O'Keefe
Copy Editor: Jane Palmer
Proofreader: Erin Geile

Dedication

This book is dedicated to my family and friends who have always believed in me and encouraged me to pursue my dreams. It is also dedicated to all my mentors who have helped shape me into the person I am today. I would not have done it without you all.

Acknowledgments

I would like to thank my husband for his support and for always allowing me room to grow into the person I am today. He sees the long nights and the hard work that goes into everything I do and yet still encourages me to fervently pursue my dreams. Thanks babe.

I would like to thank my Dean, Dr. Suzanne Prevost, who encouraged me to pursue this project. She connected me with prolific writers who helped me with various aspects of this project, including Dr. Carol Huston, who graciously walked me through my first book contract and offered invaluable insight into the book writing process. I also thank Dean Prevost for simply believing in my ability to achieve great things. Thank you.

To Dr. Safiya George, a woman who has inspired me beyond words—you are my role model. For the first time, I saw a successful scientist who looked like me and was not apologetic about who she was. Thank you for inspiring me in more ways than one and for encouraging me to have a vision for my research career.

I would also like to acknowledge a dear friend and colleague, Dr. Rebecca Martin, for her extensive expertise and knowledge that she shared with me as I was writing this book. I appreciate her support.

To Dr. Whitnee Brown, thank you for contributing Chapter 7 to this book. Thank you for your friendship and for just being eager to always jump into something with me. I appreciate your enthusiasm and support.

Many thanks go to my friends, Drs. Shirley Martin and Kristen Priddy, for their generous support in providing their experiences and insights related to othering in nursing and academia.

Susan Zulu, my Suzzeni—you convinced me that I had something important to share and the world was ready for it. Thank you for always seeing the best in me.

I would like to thank Dr. Lori Davis, the genius mentor who has taught me everything I know about building, managing, and sustaining innovative and highly productive research teams. I'm blessed to have the opportunity to learn from you. You are an incredible role model.

This book also benefits from many of my wonderful mentors and role models who have provided pearls of wisdom on how to thrive in academia. Thanks to all of you for giving of yourselves and your wisdom.

Lastly, I would love to thank all the Sigma staff who have been so gracious to me from the time this project was conceptualized to publication. Special thank yous to Ms. Emily Hatch, who has literally held my hand and offered encouragement throughout this process, and Ms. Meaghan O'Keeffe for capturing my voice so well. Carla— thank you for understanding my vision for this book and helping me bring it to reality. You are all great assets to Sigma.

About the Author

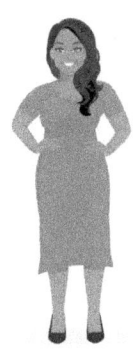

Mercy Ngosa Mumba, PhD, RN, CMSRN, FAAN, is an award-winning scientist and philanthropist. She is a published author in peer-reviewed scientific journals, and her research is widely funded by various agencies, including the National Institutes of Health (NIH). She is an Associate Professor and Founding Director of the Center for Substance Use Research and Related Conditions in the Capstone College of Nursing at the University of Alabama. She is also a Sigma liaison to the United Nations. She graduated with her PhD from the University of Texas at Arlington College of Nursing and Health Innovation in December 2016 and with her honors bachelor of science in nursing in December 2010.

Her research focuses on substance use disorders, addictive behaviors, and their comorbid mental health conditions. She is particularly interested in the impact of social determinants of health and the role of health disparities in preventing, treating, and managing these conditions. Mumba is passionate about improving the human condition through evidence-based initiatives and interventions and is a strong advocate for increasing research productivity, infrastructure, and human capital globally. She is personally involved in many initiatives that improve healthcare outcomes and promote holistic wellness and quality of life among individuals and communities worldwide. Mumba **gained tenure and was promoted from Assistant Professor to Tenured Associate Professor in a record-breaking three years.** She has $17 million in grant funding and is principal investigator on studies supported by over $9 million of extramural funding, including from the National Institutes of Health.

As an educator, she enjoys transferring knowledge to the next generation of nurse clinicians, nurse educators, nurse leaders, and nurse scientists. She is especially grateful for the opportunity to mentor the next generation of scientists, regardless of discipline and profession. She is an exceptional researcher, and her intraprofessional research lab at the

University of Alabama is home to several undergraduate and graduate honor students from various professions and disciplines, including nursing, medicine, biochemistry, psychology, public health, social work, engineering, and education. She has worked collaboratively with and mentored high-achieving students for almost 10 years. She believes that mentoring has benefits for both the mentor and mentee because it invigorates passion for inquiry and discovery.

Mumba is also a passionate servant leader who believes in the power of advocacy to effect policy changes that result in positive population outcomes. She serves on many boards and committees internationally, nationally, and locally, including the International Organization of African Nurses, the American Psychiatric Nurses Association, the Southern Nursing Research Society, and Sigma Theta Tau International's **Epsilon Omega Chapter**. She believes in giving back to the profession of nursing through service, scholarship, and mentorship. Professional engagements and service make Mumba's work worthwhile and allow her the opportunity to interact with people from all walks of life from around the world. She considers herself a global citizen, and her worldview is informed by diverse perspectives from interactions with individuals around the globe.

Every summer, Mumba takes a group of nursing students on medical mission trips to Zambia, Africa, where she was born and raised. They set up mobile clinics in rural areas, providing free healthcare services to some of the most vulnerable and disadvantaged communities in Zambia. She is especially passionate about this work because it is her way of giving back to the communities she grew up in. She also works collaboratively with the University of Zambia School of Nursing and Lusaka Apex Medical University to provide consultative services related to uptake and implementation of evidence-based nursing in both the nursing school curricula and practice settings. Mumba's long-term goal for Africa is to improve the quality of nursing education in Zambia and other African countries, increase the number of doctorally prepared nurses, and improve patient outcomes through implementation of person-centered healthcare systems and processes.

Contributing Author

Whitnee C. Brown, DNP, CRNP, FNP-C, PMHNP-BC, became a full-time Clinical Assistant Professor at the Capstone College of Nursing (CCN) at The University of Alabama in 2019. Her nursing career began in oncology, where she worked in inpatient oncology, medical oncology, gynecologic oncology, and radiation oncology. She has also worked in other areas of nursing, including medical-surgical, orthopedics, neurology, and neurology–ICU. She has worked as a nurse clinician, supporting the launch of multiple electronic health record programs. Brown has served as a preceptor for ADN-to-BSN programs, BSN programs, and MSN programs for many colleges and universities over the years.

Prior to her transition into academia, she had 10 years of nursing experience, including many leadership roles. Brown has been a family nurse practitioner for four years and continues to maintain her practice by working with a local hospitalist service as well as providing community wellness care. Her clinical expertise focuses on opioid diversion, misuse, and abuse. Brown conducts research addressing the opioid crisis, predominantly focusing on the provider's impact through the use of prescription drug monitoring program (PDMP) technology, specifically in Alabama. Her other research interests include telemedicine, informatics, rural healthcare, healthcare policy, and nurse practitioner entrepreneurship.

Brown is a member of the CCN Caring Fund Committee and Faculty Practice Council at The University of Alabama, Central Alabama Nurse Practitioner Association, Sigma Theta Tau International, Nurse Practitioner Alliance of Alabama, and Alpha Kappa Alpha Sorority. She has presented her research at the local level and at a national research conference.

Free Book Resources

To download a sample chapter, templates, and additional book resources, visit the Sigma Repository at http://hdl.handle.net/10755/22478 or navigate using the QR code below.

Table of Contents

About the Author................................ vii
Contributing Author............................. ix
Foreword....................................... xv
Introduction.................................. xix

I Welcome to Academia 1

1 Becoming an Educator 3
Three Pillars of Higher Education 4
Types of Entry-Level Academic Appointments 6
Choosing the Right Position for You 10
12-Month and 9-Month Appointments: What's the
   Difference?....................................... 13
Let's Talk Distribution of Effort (DOE) 19
Understanding the Role of an Educator................. 22
Final Thoughts 25

2 Academic Teaching Is an Art................. 27
Managing Your Workload........................... 29
Beyond Workload Units to Practicality 33
Teaching Assignment Overload 35
Confidence-Building Strategies in the Classroom 36
Evaluating Your Teaching Effectiveness................. 43
Final Thoughts 46

3 Secrets of Networking and Collaboration
in Academia 49
What Is Networking?................................ 50
Networking as an Exchange of Information.............. 53
Strategies for Creating Meaningful Networks and
   Collaborations.................................... 57
Social Media as a Networking Tool.................... 64
Strategic Classifications of Networks and Collaborations 68
Final Thoughts 71

4 Service and Academic Citizenship 73
What Is Academic Citizenship? 74
The Risk of Overcommitment. 86
Prioritizing the Right Type of Service for You 90
Final Thoughts 92

II Choosing the Best Role for You 93

5 So You've Chosen Tenure Track: Finding the Right College for You. 95
History of Tenure Track 96
Factors to Consider When Choosing a College of Nursing ... 99
Falling Behind. 109
Special Considerations for Minority and Foreign-Born Faculty 111
Final Thoughts 114

6 Becoming a Nurse Researcher and Scientist ... 115
Defining Your Program of Research 116
Developing a Strategic Plan. 119
Creating a Research and Scholarship Plan 119
Building Your Research Team. 123
You Don't Have to "Publish or Perish". 126
Seeking Additional Opportunities for Training. 131
Strategies to Maximize Grant Funding 133
Establish Yourself as a Member of Your Scientific Community 137
Evaluating Your Research and Scholarly Productivity 138
Creating a Personal Performance Improvement Plan 139
Final Thoughts 140

7 Considerations for Transitioning to a Clinical Faculty Role 141
What to Consider in Clinical Faculty Roles. 142
What Type of Organizational Environment Do You Prefer?. . . 149

　　　　Choosing a Collaborative Relationship 151
　　　　Core Competencies. 157
　　　　Specialty Considerations 159
　　　　Engaging in Research and Scholarship as a Clinical Faculty . . .161
　　　　Applying for Promotion 164
　　　　Final Thoughts 166

III　It Starts and Ends With You: Mind, Body, and Soul 167

8　Othering in Academia: An Imperative for Diversity, Equity, and Inclusion 169
　　　　Defining Othering 170
　　　　A Historical Perspective on Othering. 171
　　　　Othering in Academia 172
　　　　Intersectionality of Race and Gender 175
　　　　Race and Racism in Nursing 177
　　　　Manifestations of Othering and Racism 178
　　　　The Antidotes for Othering in Academia 190
　　　　Organizational-Level Strategies to Counter Othering in
　　　　　　Academia. 196
　　　　Individual-Level Strategies to Counter Othering in
　　　　　　Academia. 199
　　　　Final Thoughts 203

9　Stress Management 101 .205
　　　　Sources of Stress in Academia. 206
　　　　Managing Stress Related to Interpersonal Dynamics 213
　　　　Work-Life Balance to Prevent Burnout 218
　　　　Final Thoughts 221

10　Thriving in Academia 223
　　　　Resilience: The Glue That Holds Everything Together 224
　　　　Grit 231
　　　　Imposter Syndrome. 232

Mentoring..233
Formal Resilience Training 239
Final Thoughts 239

A Application Process 251

B Sample Lesson Plan 255

C Service Commitment Contact Hours..........259

References 261

Index..273

Foreword

Early in my nursing career, when I was engrossed in my critical care practice, I returned to graduate school with the goal of becoming an expert clinician. At that time, I did not aspire to, nor envision, a move into nursing education. As I gained experience, I received increasing encouragement and invitations to engage in teaching. It started with orienting and precepting new graduates, then teaching continuing education sessions for coworkers—followed by offers to supervise student clinical rotations and provide guest lectures at local colleges and conferences.

Eventually, I moved into a formal joint appointment role where my time was officially shared between a hospital and a college of nursing. After several years of shared employment, I transitioned into a full-time faculty role. I progressed through the academic ranks from assistant to associate and full professor. From there I moved into academic leadership, first in an endowed professorship, then as an associate dean, and finally to the nursing deanship I have held for nine years.

For me, the move from practice to education was a gradual transition. I progressed through my academic career with trials and errors and eventual successes, rather than following a validated series of recommendations. For many new nurse educators, this shift is more sudden and dramatic. For some, there is an element of reality shock as they discover the significant differences between nursing practice and nursing education. Whether this role change is gradual or sudden, all new nurse educators could benefit from reading a guidebook to success, such as this book.

Over the past 15 years, I have had the opportunity to recruit, hire, and mentor several novice nurse educators. Some of these nurses have adapted quickly, while others have struggled with the role transition. One of the most successful transitions I have observed is that of Dr. Mercy Mumba.

I found Mercy while I was searching LinkedIn for potential faculty prospects. At the time, I was specifically looking for nursing doctoral candidates from underrepresented groups. From my initial review of Mercy's LinkedIn profile, I could tell that she was a vibrant young nurse who was confident and committed to improving nursing practice and advancing her own career. I noticed that she had a passion for research and an uncommon degree of initiative from her list of accomplishments in her first few years as a nurse. I also sensed that she was very confident in her personal beliefs and convictions—comfortable in her own skin.

I made a "cold call" contact via email and told her that I was impressed with the work she was doing. Then I asked if she had plans for after graduation. After a brief interaction, I asked if she would consider applying and interviewing for a faculty position at our college.

That first contact was five years ago, and our college has been reaping the benefits ever since. Mercy is the consummate role model of a successful transition from nurse clinician to graduate student to accomplished teacher, scientist, and tenured faculty member. In this book, she shares powerful insights from her recent experiences as a novice educator. She also shares from her vantage point of being a very effective mentor to students, nurse clinicians, and other new educators, as well as her expertise in leading interdisciplinary teams and community service organizations.

Nursing is one of the most noble and rewarding professions, and a career in nursing education provides the perfect opportunity to increase your impact exponentially through the development of future generations of professional nurses. I trust you will find this book to be a helpful road map to a successful career transition into nursing education, and I hope you will truly enjoy this exciting journey.

–Suzanne S. Prevost, PhD, RN, FAAN
Past President, Sigma Theta Tau International Honor Society of Nursing
Nursing Professor and Angelyn Adams Giambalvo Dean
Capstone College of Nursing
The University of Alabama

Introduction

Congratulations for starting this new chapter in your professional career. For many people, this is a significant life change that can be stressful and difficult. But do not fret. In this book, we will explore strategies to help you successfully transition to academia, regardless of your reasons for pursuing an academic role.

Oftentimes, transitioning to academia may feel like starting over; this can be a source of frustration for many people because they are used to being experts in their field, and all of a sudden, they feel like novices once again. As you transition into your academic role, consider Benner's Novice to Expert Model (Benner, 2001), and cut yourself some slack. In a matter of years, you will have transitioned from a novice nurse educator to an expert nurse educator.

We say that in nursing, the possibilities are endless because there is just so much you can do with your career. I like to say that the possibilities in academia are *almost* endless because academia works a little differently. Understanding your role as an educator in your specific college or school of nursing requires understanding the mission, vision, core values, organizational structure, and strategic plan for your institution and college.

While institutions of higher learning are about the business of learning, they thrive only when structure is upheld, and everyone brings their best to the table. Think of yourself as a piece in a well-crafted puzzle. This means that you have a specific role and function, and this role is relevant in the context of the larger puzzle. Therefore, understanding your role will be informed by having a good grasp of all these dynamic aspects of your institution.

Equally important is the understanding of the culture and priorities of your institution. You have to evaluate whether your personal philosophy aligns with the philosophy of the institution prior to joining it. Otherwise, your puzzle piece may not be able to fit in the institutional puzzle, which may lead to feelings of unappreciation and, at worst, job loss. Nonetheless, most institutions of higher learning have three major focus areas: education, service, and research.

Anyone in academia will tell you that these institutions exist to educate future professionals. Therefore, being an educator is a significant responsibility in helping the institution meet its core purpose. There may be a heavy emphasis on research and scholarship depending on your type of institution, but individual expectations will vary based on the type of appointment you receive.

Whether you are coming from clinical practice, industry, the corporate world, community-based practice, or any other type of practice setting, transitioning into academia requires you to stash your proverbial toolbox with the necessary tools for the job to be effective in your new role and to quickly acclimate to this unique environment. Indeed, you may have heard some horror stories. However, this book provides you with a step-by-step guide to transitioning to an academic role. We address all things academia, and nothing is off limits.

This book is divided into three parts.

Part I: Welcome to Academia

Part I of this book is divided into four chapters. In Chapter 1, we address your role as an educator, what this means for different types of appointments, and strategies to increase your chances of success. Chapter 2 explores various aspects of teaching, including measures used to evaluate teaching effectiveness. In Chapter 3, we delve into the secrets of networking and collaboration in academia. This chapter includes a discussion on strategies for creating meaningful collaborations, maximizing your network, and growing collaborations outside of your academic unit or college. In Chapter 4, we explore the concepts of service and academic citizenship. We discuss some strategies on how to prioritize different types of service opportunities, gauge how much service is appropriate for different types of roles, and determine the implications for professional and personal growth.

Part II: Choosing the Best Role for You

Part II is divided into three chapters. Chapter 5 provides strategies and insights to choose the right college for you based on your research and scholarship objectives. From understanding college research infrastructure and support to evaluating the college culture related to research and scholarship, we address it all.

In Chapter 6, we delve into several concepts that are pertinent to your development and success as a nurse scientist, including identifying a mentor, developing a research and scholarship plan, building your team, and evaluating your productivity and the impact of your work.

In Chapter 7, we discuss considerations for clinical faculty transitioning to academia. These include tradeoffs related to salary, time, and work-life balance. We also explore various cultures related to different doctoral degree programs. Furthermore, we explore strategies to negotiate clinical practice time, possibilities for upward mobility, and everything you need to know about collaborative agreements. This chapter also examines various strategies to leverage your clinical expertise in the world of academia. We touch on community-engaged research, translational research, reflective practice, and avenues to support clinical faculty in academia.

Part III: It Starts and Ends With You: Mind, Body, and Soul

You finally made it to the last part of this book. Up to this point, we have discussed your transition to your academic role and what that entails. We have covered important concepts that have hopefully increased your understanding of academia and provided strategies that will make your transition period worthwhile and set you up for success. However, as in life in general, it is easy to get so immersed into professional growth and "making it in life." We all want to one day say, "Mama, I made it!" Right? Of course.

However, as you pursue your professional goals, we want you to always remember that there are other parts of your life that should flourish as well. Making this a reality is a personal choice that should be easier, but that is not always the case. We all have seasons when work seemingly takes over our entire lives—like it is for me right now as I am writing this book. The important thing is to find a balance and learn to intentionally attend to various aspects of your life. This may look different in each season of life. I encourage you to have goals for your personal life just the same way you have goals for your professional life. No one will take care of you for you. It all starts and ends with you.

Chapter 8 explores a very important topic for nursing and academia. We examine the history of othering in society, nursing, and academia. We also discuss the intersectionality of race and gender, and manifestations of othering, including bias, microaggression, and overt racism. Furthermore, we examine white privilege and its role in maintaining structural and systemic racism. Lastly, we provide antidotes for othering in academia, both at the organizational and individual level.

In Chapter 9, we discuss stress in academia and its sources. We also give you some tools to manage your stress and find healthy ways to cope with difficult situations. We further talk about the importance of self-care, its benefits, and falling in love with you again. Lastly, we talk about steady winning the race.

Chapter 10 introduces a number of concepts that will help you not just survive but thrive. We discuss how a change of mindset is important in building resilience and strategies to develop your self-efficacy. Part III of this book is designed to help you remember that you are a human *being*. Moreover, sometimes it is important to just *be*!

Let's Get Started

Throughout the book, you will find a recurring section titled "Mercy's Moments," where I share the many things I have learned on my own journey in academia. I share funny and sometimes even embarrassing stories to illustrate a point or emphasize a concept.

I give you a glimpse into my personal triumphs and tragedies of transitioning into an academic role, and that's OK.

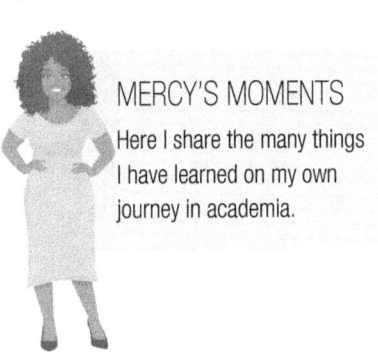

MERCY'S MOMENTS
Here I share the many things I have learned on my own journey in academia.

You'll also find "Success Nuggets" as you go along—small tidbits of information that either reinforce important points or offer additional tips.

SUCCESS NUGGET

Here I give you tidbits of information that either reinforce important points or offer additional tips.

So, hang tight, and let us equip you to not only survive academia but also thrive while you're at it. Again, welcome to academia!

–Mercy Ngosa Mumba, PhD, RN, CMSRN, FAAN

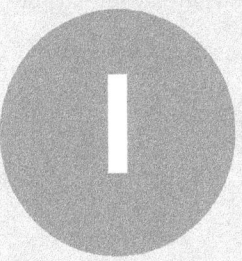

WELCOME TO ACADEMIA

1 Becoming an Educator 3

2 Academic Teaching Is an Art 27

3 Secrets of Networking and Collaboration
　in Academia 49

4 Service and Academic Citizenship 73

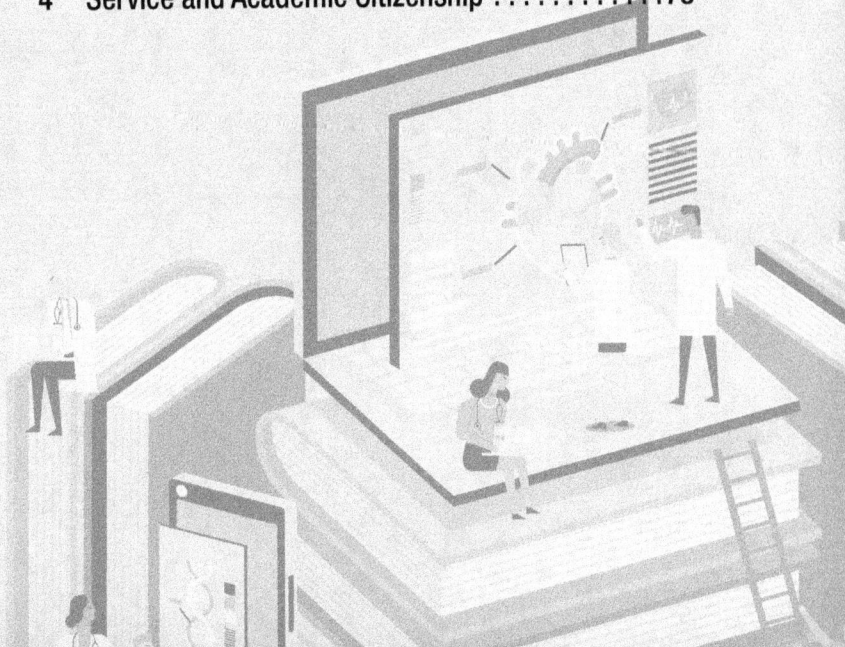

1

BECOMING AN EDUCATOR

According to Maslow's hierarchy (1943), basic physiologic needs must be met before an individual can attend to any other needs. In the expanded version (Maslow, 1970), you will notice that the classification of needs according to this hierarchy are further subdivided into two important categories—deficiency needs and growth needs. Maslow believed that the basic needs are considered deficiency needs because they arise from deprivation, and satisfying them is foundational to preventing unpleasant feelings and consequences. Growth needs, on the other hand, correspond with the highest needs on the pyramid. They represent an individual's need to grow and improve as a person and thus lead to the highest levels of self-actualization.

Similarly, as you transition into your academic role and begin to learn more about becoming an educator, there are basic deficiency needs that must be addressed prior to moving on to your growth needs. These basic needs in academia may represent your ability to understand the intricate details of the function and organizational structure of your institution and how these impact daily operations and your role as an educator.

Without this necessary foundation, it might be impossible to reach self-actualization in your academic role—or at best, it might take unnecessarily long to get to self-actualization. Therefore, in this chapter we explore the basic concepts you need to know about academia, how they relate to your role as an educator, and why understanding them is important to your successful transition.

Three Pillars of Higher Education

The three pillars of higher education are service, research and scholarship, and teaching. We address each of these in more detail later in this chapter and in other chapters as well. To summarize:

Service

The profession of nursing is encapsulated in service. Service encompasses all the activities and opportunities that individuals engage in to promote the operations of the college and institution, activities that promote nursing as a profession, and any community volunteering that promotes specific causes or outcomes. Investing time in improving conditions for others can include volunteering your time at a blood drive or holding a leadership position in a local, state, national, or international organization. Service provides the opportunity to be a change agent in the community but may also prove beneficial in assisting you to draw attention to your research and other scholarship activities.

Research and Scholarship

Research involves all the activities that lead to the generation of new knowledge in a specific field. Scholarly and other creative activities encompass all other efforts that bridge research to real world application, including disseminating of findings, translation of evidence-based practice into clinical practice, and community engagement opportunities that promote population outcomes. This is an important pillar of higher education as it improves the standing of the university and leads to sponsored programs and other funding opportunities, all of which are necessary to sustain university operations.

Teaching

The last pillar of higher education is teaching. As I mentioned in the introduction, teaching is a work of the heart and is the reason higher education exists. The type of teaching and student mentoring one can be involved in is largely based on qualifications, certifications, and institutional policies and procedures governing these decisions.

The Fourth Pillar: Administration

An aspect of academia that most people do not think about is administration. Although this is traditionally not considered a pillar of academia, it is important to note that the university or academic unit cannot function without administrators who are responsible for the day-to-day operations of the institution and are often supported by a diverse staff representing an array of expertise and functions. The administration and operations side of academia may also include other departments such as human resources.

Therefore, a successful career in academia requires a balance among these important pillars (illustrated in Figure 1.1) and a basic understanding of how your personal and professional objectives are informed by each of these pillars. Knowing this will be a prerequisite to choosing the best entry-level academic appointment for you.

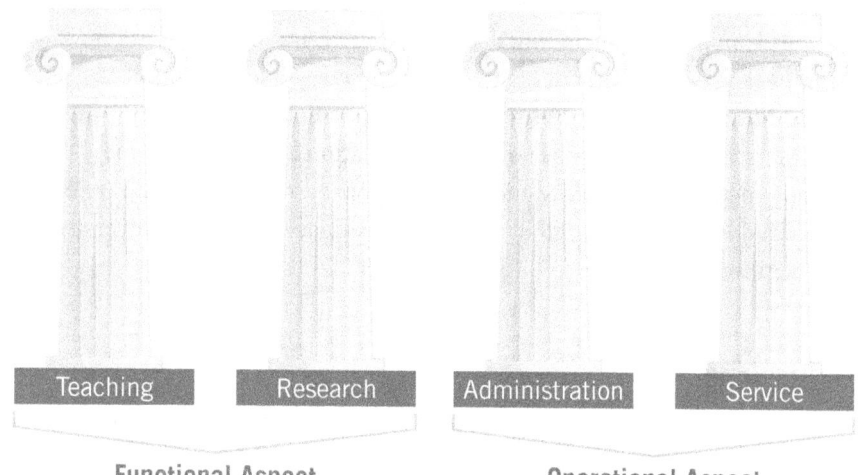

Figure 1.1 Pillars of academia.

Types of Entry-Level Academic Appointments

There are five major types of entry-level academic appointments:

- Tenure-track assistant professor
- Clinical-track assistant professor
- Instructor
- Administrative
- Adjunct

Institutions may differ in what these appointments are called, but classifications and related responsibilities and duties are generally similar across the board.

Tenure-Track Assistant Professor

Most tenure-track positions have a strong emphasis on research and scholarly productivity. There is an expectation to teach as well, but requirements for teaching vary depending on the institution. The specific roles and responsibilities of tenure-track faculty can also differ per academic institution. Nonetheless, this role is designed to lead to tenure and promotion within a specified time period if the expectations of that role are met.

Most universities require faculty to be on tenure track for about five to seven years, after which a decision must be made (mandatory decision year) whether the faculty member meets the prescribed criteria for promotion and/or tenure. These may include maintaining certain teaching benchmarks, securing external funding to support research and scholarly activities, peer-reviewed publications, and other service requirements. Sometimes, faculty members may choose to have their performance evaluated prior to their mandatory decision year if they feel they have either met or exceeded the prescribed criteria for promotion and/or tenure within their institution. Notably, sometimes faculty are promoted to a higher rank and not receive tenure or vice versa. However, in most cases, faculty will be promoted to a higher rank and receive tenure at the same time if they meet the prescribed criteria. Furthermore, tenure-track faculty are evaluated on two separate metrics annually—one is for their annual merit review like all other faculty and the other for progress toward tenure and promotion.

It is important to note that not all faculty may be allowed to begin their academic role on the tenure track. Review your university policies and procedures related to qualifications for this type of position.

For example, in some colleges of nursing, individuals with a doctor of nursing practice (DNP) terminal degree are not allowed to pursue tenure-track positions, while some colleges are able to hire DNP-prepared faculty into tenure track positions. We delve more into the nitty gritties of tenure track in Chapters 5 and 6.

Clinical-Track Assistant Professor

Clinical-track positions, on the other hand, have a greater emphasis on clinical practice and expertise as well as teaching. Faculty who are hired on clinical-track positions have a greater emphasis on and responsibility to adequately prepare students for clinical and practice roles. What courses you are assigned to teach depend on your experience and clinical background. For example, if you are a critical care nurse, you will most likely teach in critical care courses. You would not be expected to teach a mental health nursing course. Therefore, extensive clinical expertise and background are often required for these roles. Relatedly, the expectation for teaching is much higher for clinical-track faculty. Conversely, there is minimal expectation for research and scholarly productivity compared to tenure-track faculty, but it is an expectation of the role.

Clinical-track faculty may maintain a formal faculty practice, which is an additional avenue to continue practicing while maintaining their academic role as well as earn extra income. This is not mandatory for all individuals who are on the clinical track. Similar to tenure-track positions, some institutions may have restrictions on who is allowed to be in clinical-track positions based on academic preparation and/or certifications. For example, a college of nursing may have policies stipulating that only individuals with advanced practice degrees are eligible for clinical-track positions. Lastly, it is important to note that not all institutions award tenure to clinical-track professors. Therefore, if you are interested in the clinical-track role, but tenure is important to you as well, make sure you choose an institution where it is allowed. The intricacies of faculty practice are explored in Chapter 7.

Instructor Positions

Clinical instructors primarily act as clinical site supervisors and have fewer didactic teaching responsibilities. Instructors are primarily hired to take students to the clinical setting (at the undergraduate level) or to supervise other clinical experiences for graduate students (e.g., nurse practitioner students). Instructors may also have opportunities to teach didactic courses (whether online or in person); however, these opportunities may be limited depending on the institution. Depending on the program, some colleges of nursing may require a master's degree in nursing to be employed at the instructor/adjunct level, while others may require a bachelor's degree with significant clinical experience. It is also possible that individuals hired to work with primarily DNP students would be required to hold a similar doctoral degree. Although there is no requirement for research and scholarship with the instructor type of appointment, it is encouraged whenever possible.

Administrative Positions

Administrative positions have an emphasis on administrative duties related to a specific role. It is quite unlikely for entry-level academic positions to be primarily administrative positions. This is because most administrative positions require an in-depth understanding of the inner workings, policies, and procedures of an academic organization, which is often lacking for people who are first transitioning into an academic role. In a few cases, you may find that an individual is hired directly into an administrative role because they have extensive administration expertise from other roles they have held outside of academia—if that expertise is very relevant to a particular role.

Most administrative positions have a minimal expectation to teach (depending on the position), but the majority of the full time equivalent (FTE) for such a position is dedicated to administrative duties. These administrative roles may also have a concurrent classification as either clinical-track or tenure-track assistant professor. Highly qualified individuals may be hired at the associate professor level, but this is quite rare. We address this more later in the chapter when we talk about distribution of effort.

Adjunct Positions

The adjunct faculty member role is a part-time commitment, which typically implies a lesser course load and fewer teaching responsibilities. Adjunct faculty are solely focused on teaching the specific course or section of the course for which they are hired. There are no other expectations for this role. Teaching responsibilities may include, but are not limited to, student performance evaluation, office hours, course leading, curriculum development, and live or virtual instruction. The minimum requirements to qualify for this position (depending on the program in which someone is teaching) may include holding a master's degree in nursing or other health-related discipline and/or being a licensed registered nurse (RN).

Choosing the Right Position for You

With all this in mind, it is important to choose the right entry-level appointment for your academic role. The choice of which type of appointment to pursue depends on your personal career goals as well as established institutional guidelines related to qualifications. Most of the frustration in the transition period stems from a mismatch between your career objectives and the type of position you are hired into.

The type of position you are hired into—combined with your expertise, degrees, and certifications—will further dictate what type of courses you teach and how much time you are provided to focus on your research and scholarly activities. If you are primarily passionate about growing as a researcher and scientist, a tenure-track position may be best for you. On the other hand, if you are more passionate about clinical supervision of students and development of the next generation of nurse clinicians and practitioners, a clinical-track or instructor role may be your best option. At the end of the day, the most important questions revolve around what your area of expertise is, which pillar of higher education your skillset contributes to the most, and what your overall career aspirations are.

Furthermore, in some institutions, there is an unspoken and often informal hierarchy that may place tenure-track or tenured faculty at a higher rank than nontenure-track or nontenured faculty. Although this happens often in academia, it is not right. All faculty bring unique contributions to the college or institution, and this varied expertise is foundational to producing future nurse clinicians, researchers, leaders, policy experts, and public health experts. This hierarchy will differ from institution to institution. It is important to know how the degree you hold and the entry-level position you select is valued at the institution where you choose to become faculty.

These hierarchies, unfortunately, may be significant determinants for career progression, personal satisfaction with your job, and work-life balance. Therefore, it is important to understand these classifications (and the spoken and unspoken hierarchies) as they also determine the evaluation criteria used by your college for your annual merit reviews. Figure 1.2 shows the way the various positions relate to one another. Lastly, these classifications influence the criteria for promotion from one type of appointment to another. So, choose wisely.

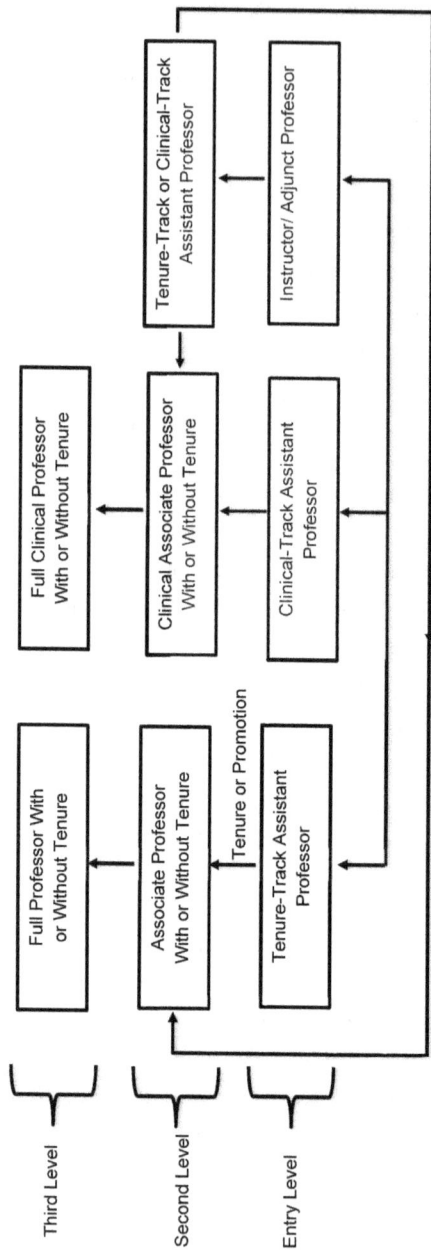

Figure 1.2 Entry-level academic positions and pathways for promotion and/or tenure.

> **SUCCESS NUGGET**
>
> The five major types of entry-level academic appointments are tenure-track assistant professor, clinical-track assistant professor, instructor, administrative, and adjunct. Choose the right appointment and institution for you based on your career goals and objectives.

12-Month and 9-Month Appointments: What's the Difference?

Another aspect to consider related to appointment types is 12-month versus 9-month appointments. These two positions are quite different, and they both have advantages and disadvantages. Most colleges like to have a good mixture of both 9-month and 12-month faculty to ensure appropriate coverage for teaching and other responsibilities in the college throughout the year.

12-Month Appointments

A 12-month appointment means that you are committed to your faculty role all year. The most significant advantage is earning approximately 30% more annually compared to a 9-month appointment. Usually with this type of appointment, you are required to teach year-round, including the summer, unless your teaching effort has been bought out or adjusted based on your research and/or other administrative duties.

You can accrue annual and sick leave as a 12-month employee. Therefore, you must formally request leave days and sick days when you are in this type of position, which is quite different from the 9-month appointment. This can sometimes be viewed as inflexible and deter people from considering 12-month appointments. Nonetheless, you still get all recognized holidays off and breaks as designated by your institution. These appointments are very common for individuals who are in administrative roles as well as some predominantly research-related positions. However, it is also quite common to see clinical faculty in these roles, especially when the college has year-round admissions that require clinical and didactic supervision of students during the summer months.

Most universities still allow faculty on 12-month appointments to have another position outside of their university appointment. However, there is a limit on how many hours of external compensation are allowed by your institution. This may also depend on the type of position you hold. For example, senior level administrators may not be allowed to hold another paid position outside of their university appointment but can be allowed to engage in certain types of consulting opportunities.

Therefore, it is important that you understand your institution's policies and procedures related to external compensation if you are going to take on a paid position outside your academic institution. This ensures that you are complying with set standards, which will help you avoid problems. Lastly, when you are on a 12-month appointment, you may be paid biweekly or monthly. Ensuring you understand the frequency of your pay will be helpful in planning for your financial responsibilities.

9-Month Appointments

A 9-month appointment simply means that you work 9 months of the year (usually coinciding with the academic year), and you are off for three months (usually coinciding with the summer months).

Advantages of 9-Month Appointments

Advantages of the 9-month appointment include being off in the summer, having more flexibility over your time, and being able to take on other jobs in the summer, if needed. This might be enticing for people who want to be in an academic setting but also want to maintain an informal clinical practice, which allows them to remain clinically relevant. As with the 12-month appointment, most institutions have limits on how much you can work outside your college or university *during the academic year*. Additionally, categories of what is counted toward this limit may vary by institution.

For example, paid consulting opportunities as well as a formal clinical position outside your university appointment might both count toward this limit. Notably, for most universities, 9-month faculty may take on paid positions in the summer months without prior approval; if the additional job is during the academic year, prior approval and disclosure are usually required. Know the policies and procedures for your institution to ensure you are functioning within the prescribed guidelines.

Additionally, 9-month appointments may be preferred if you are on tenure track because they allow the flexibility to earn a salary in the summer from grant-funding agencies to support your program of research. If you are a 9-month tenure-track faculty, you are not automatically required to teach during the summer because you are supposed to be off. This arrangement has the potential to free up about three months of the year to dedicate to growing your program of research as well as growing as a scientist.

When you are first starting your career in academia, it is quite hard to manage teaching, service, and research during the academic year, and sometimes, it's easier for your research and scholarly activities to take the back seat during the academic year. So, you may tend to play catch-up during the summer. I share more on this in Chapter 5. The good news is that if you have grant funding, you can budget your summer effort into the grant funds so that you receive summer pay for working on your research. This further increases how much you can earn while working on your research.

However, even without the opportunity to receive summer research funds, the summer may still be an opportune time to focus on research and scholarly activities. This will help you stay on track with meeting the requirements for tenure and promotion with each annual dossier review.

Another advantage of the 9-month appointment is that you can choose whether or not you want to teach summer courses. Teaching summer courses gives faculty new to an academic role the opportunity to teach an extra course or two to improve their teaching abilities, but it can also serve as another source of income for individuals on 9-month appointments. The downside is that the summer salary may be considered as supplemental income and may be taxed at a higher rate; be diligent in understanding how this works for your institution to avoid any surprises with your paycheck.

Disadvantages of 9-Month Appointments

The most important disadvantage of the 9-month appointment is the salary differential. When you opt to have a 9-month appointment, the university pays you for only 9 months instead of 12 (or 11 months if the university does not count the vacation days accrued annually as part of your working days). This gives you a conversion factor of 12 divided by 9 (1.33). For example, say your annual gross salary before taxes is $96,000 for working 12 months. When you opt to have a 9-month appointment, the university divides your 12-month salary by the conversion factor of 1.33. In this case, your 9-month salary would be $72,180.45. This makes sense because you have approximately three months off in the summer and are free to do whatever you want, including getting another job.

$$\$96,000 \div 1.33 = \$72,180.45$$

If the institution you are working for does not consider the vacation days accrued during the year, which usually equal approximately one month, as part of your working days during the year, the conversion factor for your salary will be 11 divided by 9 (1.22). Using the same figures above, your 9-month salary would be $96,000 divided by a conversion factor of 1.22. In this case, your 9-month salary would be $78,688.52.

$$\$96,000 \div 1.22 = \$78,688.52$$

As you can see from these two examples, the differences in your 9-month salary can be significant depending on whether your institution uses a 12/9 (1.33) or 11/9 (1.22) conversion factor. This is also true for instances when you want to transition to a 12-month appointment from a 9-month appointment. For example, if your 9-month salary is $75,000 annually and your institution uses a 1.33 conversion factor, your 12-month salary would be $99,750 versus $91,500 if a 1.22 conversion factor is utilized.

Salary Distribution Options for 9-month Appointments

When you are on a 9-month appointment, you have two options on how your salary can be distributed. You can opt for what is called a 9/9 disbursement plan or a 9/12 disbursement plan.

In a 9/9 plan, you opt for the university to pay your salary over the 9 months coinciding with the academic year, and you save your money to use over the three summer months that the university will not pay you. Also, when you are on a 9/9 plan, talk with someone in your institution's benefits department to make sure there are no additional considerations for your benefits package. Let's say you make $72,000 annually for your 9-month appointment. You would receive $72,000 divided by 9, or $8,000 gross salary each month for 9 months of the year (coinciding with the academic year), and you would not get paid by your institution in the summer.

Opting for the 9/12 disbursement plan means that you are choosing to have your 9-month salary redistributed over 12 months. Based on our example, this would mean getting paid $72,000 divided by 12, or $6,000 gross salary per month for all 12 months of the year. With this type of disbursement, the university withholds a certain amount each month from your 9-month monthly salary in what is called deferred pay. The university then uses the money they "held" for you during the academic year as deferred pay to pay you in the summer. Remember, this a very simplified way of illustrating this option, and it may look a little different depending on whether you get paid biweekly or monthly. Additionally, there may be caps on salaries that can opt for 9/12 disbursement plans. Make sure to speak with your institution's payroll representatives to understand the tax implications of this option.

It is important to understand these distinctions, especially for individuals who start their academic positions in the spring semester. You need to adequately plan for summer expenses if you are on a 9-month appointment (whether 9/9 or 9/12).

Special Considerations

Sometimes faculty may be allowed to have a joint appointment between their academic institution and a clinical or industry partner. In these types of arrangements, there are special considerations related to how the FTE is allocated between the two institutions. There is usually a requirement to also sign a memorandum of understanding that specifically stipulates the terms of the joint appointment. The faculty member should be careful to consider how this joint appointment may affect benefits, ability to earn tenure and promotion, salary differences, and accrual of years toward retirement.

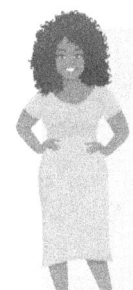

MERCY'S MOMENTS

My own story is funny today, but I promise you it wasn't funny at all when it happened! I started my 9-month academic position in the spring semester, and I did not understand the concept of deferred pay for the 9/12 plan. It also didn't help much that I started in February. I was coasting along enjoying my work and learning more about my role as an educator when suddenly my May paycheck hit my bank account. Poor me thought payroll made a mistake! As oblivious as I was and with the purest of intentions, I proceeded to call my payroll department to let them know there was a mistake on my paycheck. Surely they had forgotten to include the rest of my salary.

The woman in the payroll department was so polite. She said, "Ms. Mumba, there hasn't been a mistake. You are on a 9/12 appointment, and you started in February. That means over the last two months, only $xx have been kept for you as deferred pay. This will be equally divided into three months to cover your summer salary. This means that over the next three months, your salary will be $xx/month."

Imagine my shock—I'm laughing now, but it wasn't funny then. I wasn't some rich person with major savings who just graduated from her PhD program. So yeah, my husband and I definitely had to have *the* conversation! Thankfully, I had signed up to teach some summer courses, and we had other income coming in, which proved to be very helpful in keeping our finances on track that summer.

I share this story because in my conversations with other people, I have learned that I was not alone in this blissful ignorance, which can easily lead to financial instability without proper planning. Even for the most financially stable, this situation can bring frustration. Because of this and the potential for misunderstanding, I personally caution against starting your academic appointment in the spring semester if you are on a 9-month appointment.

Let's Talk Distribution of Effort (DOE)

Let's now move on to a slightly different concept—distribution of effort (DOE). Regardless of the type of your appointment, most individuals will be required to teach a course or a section of a course in addition to expectations for research and service. How many courses one teaches varies based on several factors, including:

- Type of position (e.g., clinical track versus tenure track)
- Administrative responsibilities
- Research responsibilities
- Significant service responsibilities
- The program in which the individual teaches

Unfortunately, most people, including me, never bothered to ask about this very important issue before starting an academic role. However, this is becoming an increasingly important aspect of recruitment for many colleges of nursing and institutions everywhere. The younger generation of faculty want to know exactly what their DOE will be prior to even accepting a position (as it should be). I must say that some institutions are quite transparent about DOE and even include this verbiage in their offer letters, and others are not as clear.

Sometimes institutions are not clear about this concept mainly because they want to have the flexibility to change how effort is allocated, depending on the needs of the college and individual faculty performance. There are pros and cons to each type of scenario. However, it is still important to have a clear understanding of the breakdown of duties and responsibilities based on your position.

DOE in its truest sense can be a complex concept. In its most simple form, DOE refers to the proportion of time allocated to each major component of one's job description.

For example, someone in a tenure-track position may have the following DOE:

- 60% research and scholarship
- 30% teaching
- 10% service and academic citizenship

Simply, this means that in a 40-hour workweek, about:

- 24 hours will be dedicated to research and scholarly activities
- 12 hours will be dedicated to teaching and student advising
- 4 hours will be dedicated to service and academic citizenship

Another way to look at this would be the weight associated with the different roles and responsibilities that come with your position. This is because your DOE will also serve as the basis for expectations for your annual merit review.

This breakdown will differ based on the different types of appointments, but it should provide guidance on where and how you should exert the most energy during your workweek. It also provides guidance on how much time should be allocated to each aspect of your job.

For individuals in administrative positions, there may be a fourth category related to administrative duties. Their DOE may be as follows: 30% research and scholarly activity, 30% administrative duties, 30% teaching, and 10% service and academic citizenship.

DOE provides insight into the evaluation criteria and what weight is associated with each component of your job. DOE does not mean that you give your best only to the aspect of your job that has the highest distribution, to the neglect of others. A lot of people fall into this trap, which leads to underperformance in some aspects of their job and inadvertently affects their overall performance as a faculty member. Therefore, you still need to give 100% to each aspect of your job; you just have to be smarter about what the expected outputs in each category are, based on established policies and procedures at your institution.

For example, just because your position is 60% research, 30% teaching, and 10% service doesn't mean that you should only pay attention to meeting your research and scholarship requirements and neglect being a good teacher. You still need to have to meet established benchmarks for teaching effectiveness in your college and have a well-rounded service portfolio to satisfy evaluation criteria for your college or institution. Therefore, think of DOE as pertaining more to *quantity of expectations* and not *quality of outputs*. Figure 1.3 shows a sample distribution of effort calculation.

SUCCESS NUGGET

Work smarter, not harder: Plan your workweek based on your DOE for your type of appointment. This will set you up for success in the long run.

Understanding the Role of an Educator

Now that we understand some basic principles (the deficiency needs, according to Maslow), the question remains: What does a nurse educator do? It sounds like a simple question, but successfully transitioning into a nursing academic role requires us to understand the specific roles, duties, and responsibilities of a nurse educator. These responsibilities and duties may look different depending on the type of appointment, the program in which you are teaching, and the type of courses you are teaching.

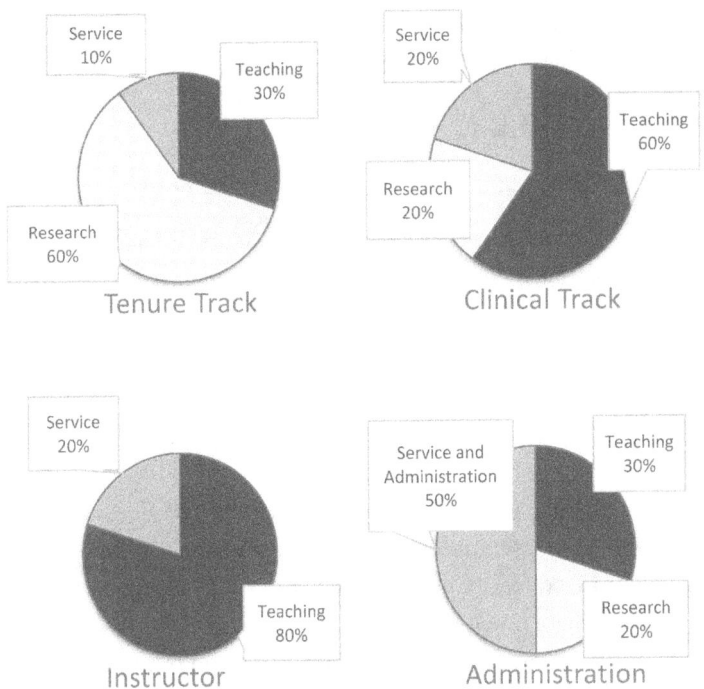

Figure 1.3 Sample DOE for various entry-level positions.

For example, your teaching approach may vary depending on whether you are teaching undergraduate or graduate students, teaching via in-class lecture or a completely online program, or teaching a didactic versus a clinical course. While there is no way to understand every detail about what your role will entail from the beginning, it is important to have a basic understanding of the college's teaching expectations for someone in your type of position.

A *nurse educator* can be defined as an individual who designs, implements, and evaluates educational curriculum for nursing and can serve as an advisor or role model to students (RegisteredNursing.

org, 2021). Based on this definition, the nurse educator role can be divided into five basic components:

- Designing and developing nursing curriculum
- Implementing nursing curriculum (i.e., teaching)
- Evaluating nursing curriculum and students' learning outcomes
- Advising students in academic and professional progression
- Serving as a role model for professional etiquette and achievement

These responsibilities may carry different weights at different times of the semester. For example, at the beginning of the semester, you may be more concerned with ensuring that your lectures are updated, your syllabi and course schedules are correct and congruent, and students understand the learning objectives and outcomes. In the middle of the semester, you may focus more on helping struggling students, mentoring students professionally, maintaining engagement with thriving students, and evaluating progress. At the end of the semester, you may concentrate more on remediating failing students and finalizing grades. And sometimes, you may have to balance several of these aspects of being an educator all at once. We explore this further in Chapter 2.

The important thing is to know when to focus on each of these roles to ensure students' success. As I mentioned earlier, institutions of higher learning are in the business of education. Therefore, at the end of the day, meeting student learning outcomes is of paramount importance.

Final Thoughts

There are many aspects that go into being an educator outside of teaching your students. Having a basic understanding of your role, your institution, and academia in general will help make your transition a smooth one. This will set you up to pursue your growth needs once you get more comfortable in your role. Be sure to ask the critical questions as you explore your teaching options, and take your time before choosing an institution. It *does* matter where you start.

2

ACADEMIC TEACHING IS AN ART

Academic teaching is an art, and success as a nurse educator is contingent on many factors. It is important to know that not everyone who transitions into academia has specific preparation in education or curriculum development. Therefore, making sure that you understand your teaching requirements is one of the first things you need to do. Also, find out what resources are available at your institution to help novice educators learn more about the educator role and curriculum development, implementation, and evaluation.

Many people think that teaching is easy. Nurses teach their patients all the time, right? Right! But academic teaching is very different from informational teaching experiences you may have had in the past. I like to say that academic teaching is an art; it takes time and intentionality to get good at it. This means that in the beginning, you will need to invest time in growing and perfecting this art. Notice that I used the word *invest*, which means to devote one's time, effort, or energy to a particular undertaking with the expectation of a worthwhile result (Oxford English Dictionary, n.d.-a). Just like most things in life, you will get out what you put in.

In fact, the first few weeks and perhaps even months of transitioning will require time, energy, and effort specifically dedicated to perfecting your art of teaching. In Chapter 1, we talked about Distribution of Effort (DOE). Assume that at first, most of your time will go to perfecting your art of teaching, regardless of your type of appointment—with the possible exception of someone in a predominantly administrative role, which is rarely an entry-level appointment for novice educators. Becoming a successful, competent educator takes time, so be patient with yourself and have a realistic expectation of what this process will look like.

SUCCESS NUGGET

Before you accept a position at an institution, find out what resources are available to help novice educators. Academic teaching is an art, and it takes time, energy, and resources to perfect the art.

MERCY'S MOMENTS

When I first started my tenure-track position, I was excited just to have a job and to begin doing what I love—research. Although I was a graduate teaching assistant (GTA) during my PhD program and worked as an adjunct instructor for two semesters, I did not realize that transitioning into a full-time role would be significantly different. I thought, I've got this—been there, done that! I did not realize how a full-time role would significantly affect how much time it would take to prepare my lessons, respond to student questions, and teach the classes. Also, I took students to the clinical site twice every week. In my mind, that was only two days a week, so I had three other days to do everything else in the world. But I did not account for the fact that I needed to provide my students with office hours, and I still needed to study and prepare for my classes. Oh, and there are meetings too! Remember that part called service and academic citizenship?

I found myself in a loop of taking students to clinical, preparing for classes, teaching classes, having office hours, and attending meetings. Then on the weekends, if I wasn't too tired, I might write a few paragraphs of a manuscript that I needed to complete. This, of course, got easier over time, and I found more time to work on my research because most of my lessons were updated after a few semesters. My point in this story is to tell you not to underestimate how much time it will take for you to transition and feel comfortable in your new role. If you don't have a realistic expectation of what this phase will look like, you may begin to feel frustrated or fear that other parts of your job are suffering. In my case, I started feeling like I was not dedicating enough time to growing my research and developing as a scientist.

After that first semester, I knew I had to do something differently. In retrospect, that initial feeling of dropping the ball in some areas of my job stemmed from not understanding the concept of DOE and not knowing how workload was calculated in my college. So, if you feel like you are stuck in this loop of barely making it because you can't manage all aspects of your job, or you want to have a smooth transition into your academic role once you take that first position, I share some strategies in the next sections that might help.

Managing Your Workload

To successfully transition into the educator role, you need to manage your workload and understand how it is calculated. For example, your institution might say that 12 units or credit hours per semester constitute a full-time teaching load, and based on your institution, this may correspond with 0.8 FTE. Different course classifications may be assigned corresponding units, which are then utilized to calculate the teaching load.

Courses may correspond with different workload units based on multiple factors. These factors include:

- The number of students in the course
- Whether the course is a theory, clinical, or combination course
- The number of faculty teaching in that course (e.g., one faculty versus three faculty members)
- In-person or online course
- Undergraduate versus graduate courses
- Serving on a dissertation committee versus chairing the dissertation committee
- Whether the course has a writing (W) designation

Table 2.1 shows an example of what an educator's workload might look like. Let's say teaching one section of a theory course with 30 students or fewer is worth three units, taking one clinical group of six to eight students (at two eight-hour clinical days per week) is six units, and serving as primary advisor to a DNP student is who is currently working on their DNP project is one unit. If you are assigned one clinical group (at two eight-hour clinical days per week), two sections of a theory course (with 30 students per section), and two DNP students who are currently working on their DNP projects, that would be considered an overload because you are at 14 hours or units, instead of the 12 hours or units stipulated by your institution as a full-time teaching load. It is important to note that in many colleges of nursing, supervision of doctoral students is not considered part of teaching workload, but rather part of service to the profession and the institution. Therefore, make sure you understand how your institution categorizes this type of work.

TABLE 2.1 CALCULATING TEACHING LOAD

Course type	Associated Units	Total
One clinical group	6 units/clinical group	6 units
Section of a theory course	3 units/section x 2 sections	6 units
Primary advisor DNP student	1 unit/student x 2 students	2 units
Total workload units		14 units

Another important aspect of understanding workload is knowing how your workload corresponds with your DOE based on the position you are in. The expectation for number of hours or units that you are required to teach will be based on your assigned DOE. For instance, if you are a clinical-track faculty and your DOE stipulates that 60% of your FTE is dedicated to teaching, then a full-time teaching load for you would be nine units. Anything more than nine units would be considered an overload for your predetermined DOE. Therefore, your teaching workload should always reflect your DOE allocation for teaching.

If 12 units = 0.8 FTE, then 0.6 FTE (60% teaching) = (12 x 0.6) / 0.8 = 9 units.

On the other hand, we know that there is a shortage of nursing faculty (American Association of Colleges of Nursing [AACN], 2020a), and sometimes administrators may need to assign more than the established teaching load to some faculty members based on the needs of the college. Best practice for assigning teaching overload is that the supervising administrator has a conversation with the affected faculty member, explaining why the college is considering assigning the additional workload, how the faculty member will be provided with the necessary resources and support to safely take on the additional teaching assignment, any adjustments to other responsibilities (e.g., research and service expectations) that will be made to accommodate the teaching overload, and how future teaching assignments will be adjusted based on the proposed overload. Unfortunately, this doesn't always happen.

In the instance where you are assigned a teaching overload and your supervising administrator has not explained the reason for the overload and adjustments that can be made to other assignments, it is your responsibility as the affected faculty member to initiate these conversations. Approach these conversations with an attitude of collaboration and problem-solving. Make sure your supervisor understands that you are willing to be a team player, but you would also like to know how adjustments in expectations for other aspects of your job will be made. This is important to ensuring that you are adequately supported as a new faculty member and not setting yourself up for failure. For example, you can negotiate to have the required number of college meetings you attend reduced to only include those necessary to your specific role. You also want to ensure that there is clear guidance on how future assignments may be adjusted based on you taking on the additional teaching load.

It is important to be flexible to help meet the needs of the college every now and again. However, be careful that you are not caught up in a perpetual cycle of teaching overload, especially if your type of appointment is focused not only on teaching, if other forms of compensation are not provided, or if you are not able to negotiate the removal of other responsibilities from your job description when you consistently take on extra teaching loads.

Inability to manage recurring teaching overloads can lead to burnout and other health problems. We talk about self-care and prioritizing mental health in the last part of this book, but I would like to emphasize that we should not normalize burnout in academia, most of which is associated with feelings of inability to manage teaching workloads. Unfortunately, due to a severe shortage of nursing faculty, this has been the norm for a while and was exacerbated by the COVID-19 pandemic (Flaherty, 2020).

Remember that student outcomes are also affected when you are consistently overloaded because you are not able to give them your best. Over time, this may lead to feelings of inadequacy and has the potential to diminish your self-efficacy in your role as an educator. If you don't know how to calculate your required workload, you might end up with a teaching overload and find yourself wondering why you can't seem to catch a break. Be careful not to associate the occasional dropping of the ball with personal deficiency.

> **SUCCESS NUGGET**
>
> It is not selfish to want an equitable teaching load. To advocate for yourself, you must know how to calculate your teaching load based on your institution's policies. When necessary, negotiate how your supervisor will adjust expectations and requirements for other aspects of your job and how future assignments will be modified to reflect the current overload.

Beyond Workload Units to Practicality

But it isn't just about the workload units—it's also about the practicality of the teaching assignment based on the type of courses you are assigned. This is often overlooked because on paper, it can still look like a fair teaching assignment based on the workload units.

Let's say you are an instructor whose DOE is 80% teaching and therefore corresponds with 12 units of teaching workload per semester. You have one clinical group (at two eight-hour clinical days per week) and two theory courses, each of them meeting three hours a day on two separate days of the week. You are required to have specified office hours for your students (at four hours per week), and you have to attend work meetings. This is an equitable assignment based on the number of workload units, which is 12 in this case.

TABLE 2.2 TEACHING LOAD PRACTICALITY

Course type	Associated Units	Total
One clinical group	6 units/clinical group	6 units
Two theory courses	3 units/course x 2 courses	6 units
Total workload units		12 units

However, because of the types of courses you are teaching and the service requirements for your college (e.g., attending required faculty meetings that may be scheduled on different days of the week), this teaching assignment and the other associated responsibilities pretty much take up Monday to Friday, with only small pockets of time left over. Notably, because you are an advanced practice registered nurse (APRN), you may be expected to dedicate a day to faculty practice, which is essential for you to maintain advanced practice certifications.

With this schedule, you are automatically forced to conduct your faculty practice on the weekends, which may negatively impact your work-life balance in the long run. In this case, the teaching assignment is not unfair nor is it considered overload, but the practicality of doing everything related to your role in a five-day workweek is quite low. And over time, this type of arrangement may become unsustainable due to chronic stress.

It's always important to have a great relationship with your supervisor, but I specifically bring this up here because having open, honest communication might help your supervisor see that your current assignment is fair but may not be practical, based on how the courses you are assigned are structured and taught. Sometimes supervisors may not be aware of how teaching assignments realistically play out and affect other aspects of your job. If you properly communicate these concerns, your supervisor may be able to reassign you to a different course that allows you to have more flexibility in your time and how your teaching responsibilities are carried out. But if not, at least they would be aware of your situation, and perhaps accommodations can be made for other responsibilities.

SUCCESS NUGGET

Having a great relationship with your supervisor provides the opportunity to have open and honest conversations when you have job-related needs that may require accommodation from your supervisor.

Teaching Assignment Overload

What I often see happen is that people who are new to academia take on teaching overload assignments without registering their concerns because they are afraid of being considered whiners. So, they suffer in silence and cannot give their best to any part of their job because they feel they are juggling multiple balls at any given time. It is often too late before anyone recognizes that this person is struggling. Sometimes these issues are discovered only during the annual evaluation, when the faculty member must provide reasons for underperformance in one or more aspects of the job. Waiting to address these concerns during the annual merit review might be too late to remedy the situation, which may cause frustration and contribute to the high faculty attrition rates seen in academia (Bucklin et al., 2014).

Most faculty members who leave academia exit within the first three years (Bucklin et al., 2014), usually because they:

- Are overwhelmed with their teaching assignments
- Experience a lack of inclusiveness
- Do not have a relationship with their supervisor or institution grounded on respect and open communication
- Lack resources and support, such as professional development for new faculty transitioning into their academic role
- Perceive that department chairs do not foster an environment for teaching, research, and service

These cited reasons for people leaving their jobs in academia have nothing to do with lack of passion for teaching or unwillingness to support their students. Therefore, if you are experiencing any of these issues, you do not have to suffer in silence and alone. Be proactive and identify a teaching mentor early in the process of transitioning into the academic role. And remember, even if you did not start out with a mentor, it is never too late for you to correct course.

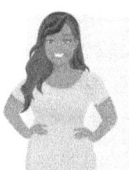

MERCY'S MOMENTS

I was fortunate to be assigned a first-year mentor when I started my full-time tenure-track position. To this day, she is one of my closest colleagues because we built a great relationship in which she allowed me to be vulnerable and ask all the "stupid" questions. She held my hand through my entire first year and took me under her wing. She familiarized me with the courses I was assigned to teach, showed me how different courses work, helped me with lesson plans, and allowed me to shadow her before I gave my first solo lecture. When I started giving solo lectures, she gave me feedback on what I did well and what I could do better. She even provided me with additional strategies to engage students during lecture. This was the best thing that could have happened to me in terms of transitioning into a full-time teaching role. That is why I am a staunch advocate for you to have a teaching mentor at your chosen institution in your first year.

Confidence-Building Strategies in the Classroom

As you can see, a lot goes into the teaching environment before you even step into the classroom. As you transition to teaching students, it is important to note that whether you are teaching in person or online, it takes time to build your comfort level.

With the increase in the number of online programs, new faculty may think it is easier to teach online than in person. This is not necessarily true. Faculty members who teach online are still expected to use interactive teaching strategies and keep students engaged with their coursework.

Becoming comfortable with delivering content to students can take time, even for the most confident person. Building confidence in teaching will stem from the knowledge that you have adequately prepared for your course. Students always have questions, and if you are not prepared, they will know. This does not mean that you will always have the answer to their questions; it means that you are able to provide accurate, up-to-date, and relevant content to your students. You have heard the familiar saying—failure to prepare is preparing to fail.

If you cannot answer your students' questions, it is OK to tell them you would be happy to investigate the issue. This is much better than providing wrong information that you will have to retract later, which can cause your students to lose trust and confidence in you as a teacher.

SUCCESS NUGGET

Your students will know when you are not well-prepared for class. Oops! And if you don't know the answer to their questions, you are better off saying so and offering to investigate. Do not overexplain your way into a hole of misinformation.

Refine Your Teaching Philosophy

A *teaching philosophy* is defined as a reflective and introspective statement of what you believe about teaching and learning and your specific strategies on how your teaching objectives can be achieved (Cornell University, 2022; O'Neal et al., 2019; Western University Centre for Teaching and Learning, n.d.). Having a great understanding of your teaching philosophy will serve as a road map to the type of educator you will become.

A teaching philosophy also provides a blueprint for how you relate to your students, what evaluation strategies you use, and how you deliver lectures. There are various philosophies on teaching, and they are often influenced by educational learning theories. Examples of educational learning theories that might influence your personal teaching philosophy include social cognitive theory, experiential learning theory, theory of human motivation, and behaviorism. While you can learn from other people, it is important to understand your own philosophy because it serves as a foundation for everything you do and provides guidance on how to resolve moral or ethical dilemmas related to your role as an educator. To learn more, I recommend reading Zhou and Brown's second edition (2015) on educational learning theories.

Educational learning theories are also usually grouped into five major categories: behaviorism, cognitivism, constructivism, humanism, and connectivism.

Behaviorism is based on the notion that behavior and knowledge are acquired through interactions with the environment, and therefore, teachers have the opportunity to directly influence behavior and knowledge acquisition in their classrooms.

Cognitivism is based on the notion that students are able to process information received from teachers and make informed choices rather than merely responding to the environmental stimuli. Therefore, in cognitivism, the students are active participants in their learning.

Constructivism is based on the notion that prior experiences and knowledge influence learning of new ideas and concepts. Therefore, in this theory, students are not simply blank slates that can receive new information and modify behavior based on environmental stimuli. Rather, new knowledge is incorporated with prior experiences to form new learning experiences, which are supposed to be richer than simply processing the new knowledge outside of the context of prior experiences.

Humanism is based on the notion that student learning is motivated by self-actualization needs. Therefore, teachers should provide a learning environment that takes care of the basic needs of the student to foster their ability to pursue self-actualization.

Connectivism is based on the notion that students will learn when they create meaningful connections with each other and other roles and obligations that have personal meaning and value. Therefore, teachers should strive to create these connections and relationships for their students to facilitate their learning.

Evaluating which educational learning theories best align with your personal values and beliefs about student learning is important in informing the development of your personal teaching philosophy. It is perfectly OK to draw from all major categories of educational learning theories or even just a few. The idea is to ensure that your teaching philosophy is broad enough to cater to different student populations but focused enough to provide you with a blueprint for your teaching.

The University of Minnesota Center for Education and Innovation has a wonderful seminar on crafting your personal teaching philosophy as well as examples of teaching philosophies by individuals representing various disciplines (2021). Additionally, the University of Michigan Center for Research on Learning and Teaching provides several tools to develop your teaching philosophy (O'Neal et al., 2019). I would highly recommend using these resources to guide the development of your personal teaching philosophy and how to evaluate its consistent implementation throughout your work as an educator.

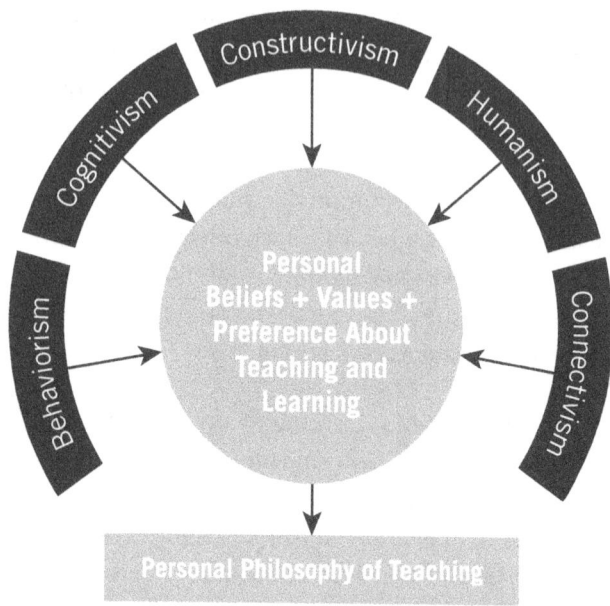

Figure 2.1 Educational learning theories influencing teaching philosophy.

Observe Seasoned Colleagues

Find seasoned colleagues who teach courses similar to yours. This will provide you with insight into the student population at your institution, ideas for keeping students engaged, and various teaching styles that you can learn and incorporate into your own. Shadowing other faculty members also introduces you to students before you have to teach them. This provides familiarity and potential interactions with students before you engage with them for the first time in your classroom as a faculty member.

Use Lesson Plans

Lesson plans are very important, especially when starting out, as they will help you stay on track when teaching. They can also prove helpful in planning your interactive activities for those long classes, especially in undergraduate nursing programs. When you first start teaching, it is easy to either rush through content and not use all the class time allocated to your course—or to do the opposite, which is to lose the structure of the class and veer off topic, making you run overtime. Both scenarios diminish your students' confidence in your ability to help them meet their learning objectives. When you plan out your class, you will be more confident in teaching your students and maximizing class time to meet students' learning objectives.

A sample lesson plan is provided in Appendix B, and is also available as a downloaded, reuseable file via the Sigma Repository at http://hdl.handle.net/10755/22478.

Adapt (With Permission) the Prior Instructor's Work

Here's one of my favorite strategies: When you are new to your role, there is no need to reinvent the wheel. Most of the time, you will start a new academic position only a few weeks before the semester begins. You may find that you will teach several lectures and possibly multiple courses. You do not have time to build all your content from scratch within this short time frame. So what can you do? Perhaps you should ask colleagues who previously taught your course for permission to modify their content for the first semester. You will have many opportunities to create and revise content as you grow as an educator. You just don't have to do it all at once. Sometimes new faculty members are overwhelmed before they even start because of this issue. The most important thing is to acknowledge during your lectures that your materials were adapted from your colleagues. Give credit where it is due, and you will be just fine.

Practice by Giving Guest Lectures

Ask your colleagues if you can provide some guest lectures for their courses. The more opportunities you have to teach, the more confident and comfortable you will be in your role as an educator. I recommend guest teaching in a variety of formats to widen your experience. For example, if you currently teach an in-person didactic course, you may seek opportunities to guest lecture in a completely online class or a class with a clinical component.

Doing so makes you versatile and increases your opportunity to grow as an educator within your college. Additionally, seeking guest-lecturing opportunities outside your college will help promote interprofessional education, and you can slowly establish yourself as a collaborator with faculty members outside your discipline.

Find a Mentor

Identifying a mentor is important for ensuring success (Baxley et al., 2014) and more so when you first transition into an academic role. This person can be inside or outside your institution. Some organizations have a more formalized mentorship program where they assign a more seasoned faculty member to serve as a mentor during a faculty member's first year. First, you may want to ask your supervisor if your college has such a program. If a formal matching process does not exist, ask your supervisor for recommendations on who would be a great person to approach.

The role of first-year mentors is to help new faculty members acclimate to the environment, explain policies and procedures, and introduce them to other faculty to help them grow their network. First-year mentors can also help new faculty understand the student population, clarify expectations for the role, and provide guidance related to teaching responsibilities and other aspects of the job.

You will read more about mentoring in Chapter 10.

> **SUCCESS NUGGET**
>
> Strategies for increasing your comfort level in the classroom include adopting a teaching philosophy, shadowing seasoned colleagues, using lesson plans to organize your class time, getting permission from colleagues to initially use their course materials, and delivering guest lectures both inside and outside your college. Consistently using these strategies will increase your self-efficacy in your educator role and may serve as a catalyst for expediting your growth and development in your academic role.

Evaluating Your Teaching Effectiveness

Now that we have discussed all the fun ways to increase your comfort in the classroom, let's move on and talk about a topic that most people do not enjoy—evaluations. As with every job, when you transition into academia, you will be evaluated on several metrics. One of them is your teaching effectiveness, which can be evaluated through various means. It is important for you to understand how your college evaluates teaching effectiveness and the policies and procedures that apply.

Student Opinion of Instructor (SOI) Scores

Some colleges only look at what are called student opinion of instructor (SOI) scores. In case you are not familiar with SOI scores, students receive a survey at the end of each semester with questions about the way your course is run. They are asked to rate you as the instructor and the course on various issues. For example, where I currently work, the instructor is evaluated on:

- Preparedness for class
- Effectiveness of communication
- Accessibility to students outside the classroom
- Overall rating of the instructor

The course is evaluated on whether or not:

- Course objectives were clearly stated
- Procedures for grading were fair
- The students thought the course was a valuable experience
- The students received the grade they anticipated in the course
- Assignments enabled the student to meet the course objectives as stated in the syllabus

The course evaluation also includes an overall course rating measured on a 5-point Likert scale, ranging from strongly agree to strongly disagree.

Knowing how you will be evaluated will help ensure that you are addressing all the categories during the course of the semester. When you know these criteria, you are better able to communicate expectations with your students while intentionally and proactively reinforcing how you are meeting these various metrics in your courses. Additionally, you should find out if there are established benchmarks for SOI scores for your college. Some may say the benchmark is 4.0/5.0 for each course, while others may consider 3.5/5 acceptable. Knowing these benchmarks will provide insight on what standards are acceptable for your college.

Although you may always want to have 5.0/5.0 for your SOI scores, this is not a realistic goal. Student opinions of instructors are just that—opinions. While they carry weight in your evaluation process, always review them with the understanding that several factors will influence how students evaluate you. Some are within your control and others are not.

Consumer research has consistently shown that there are two types of customer reviews: from very satisfied customers and very dissatisfied customers. Think of your students as customers who are reviewing your services (teaching). Sometimes these reviews are glowing, and sometimes they are not. What's important is to show a pattern of improvement and consistent attention to feedback from semester to semester. Your supervisor wants to know that you take the feedback from students seriously and are implementing strategies to fix issues that are genuinely of concern.

MERCY'S MOMENTS

I was born and raised in Zambia, Africa. When I started teaching, some students commented on my SOI report that they couldn't understand my accent. This may be a valid concern, but I can't do much about how I speak. So, I made it a habit at the beginning of the semester to tell my students that I have an accent, and I want to make sure they are successful in my course.

I welcome them to raise their hands and ask me to repeat myself if there is something they don't understand. I normalized the situation and made it OK for them to ask me to repeat myself and ask questions in class. Since then, I have not received any comments about my accent. Yes, your students want to know that you consider them and their issues as legitimate, even though you can't always solve the problem. They want to know that you hear them and are not dismissing their requests.

Trusted Faculty Feedback

Another way to evaluate your teaching effectiveness is to ask a more seasoned faculty member to attend your lecture and provide feedback on your teaching style, content delivery, student engagement strategies, and any other area the person may feel is necessary. Some institutions have a more formalized process for this peer-review evaluation. Find out if this is the case for your institution and, if so, follow the applicable policies or procedures. For example, your institution may require two peer-review evaluations of teaching effectiveness per merit review cycle. My advice is that you allow yourself to receive peer review even if it is not a requirement for your college. Feedback is always a blessing. We all have blind spots, and others may see a situation differently. Feedback helps us improve and grow.

Student Performance

Another way to evaluate your teaching is to examine how students perform on your exams, quizzes, or other assignments. While several factors contribute to student performance, teacher effectiveness is of major importance. Evaluating your teaching is particularly important when you have made significant changes to your courses or content areas. Sometimes you may want to make changes to your teaching methods because you notice that students are struggling in a specific aspect of your course or content. Other times you may ask students to provide honest feedback about a certain change and whether they perceive that teaching innovation has contributed to their success.

The most important point is to understand that your teaching effectiveness can be evaluated in various ways—be proactive in seeking feedback so that you don't have any surprises during your annual merit evaluations.

Final Thoughts

Academic teaching is truly an art. As you transition into your role as an educator, be mindful of all the different things you can do to improve your abilities. This is especially important if you do not have any formal training to be an educator (e.g., a master's degree in nursing education or a doctor of education degree). Additionally, be proactive in receiving help from trusted colleagues when you need it. You will find that creating a community of colleagues with whom you can consult on various issues as you acclimate to your role will be essential for your successful transition. I like to say that not everyone is a natural teacher, but with passion, enthusiasm, and the right resources and mentors, we can all learn the art of teaching.

3

SECRETS OF NETWORKING AND COLLABORATION IN ACADEMIA

In Chapters 1 and 2, we covered many of the nuances of transitioning into an academic role by dissecting the infrastructure of academia. Most of us take the first few months of transitioning to an academic role to concentrate on our role as an educator. While this is commendable, I often caution people not to take too long to start networking and building collaborative relationships in their new place of employment.

I mentioned earlier that I'm originally from Africa. We have an African proverb that says if you want to go fast, go alone, but if you want to go far, go together. I don't think I can find a better illustration of the importance of networking and collaboration in academia. If you want to have lasting impact in your field, you must build collaborations with various types of people. In this chapter, we explore the secrets of networking and collaborations in academia, so hang tight.

What Is Networking?

It is often said that although there are official hierarchies in academia, informal hierarchies are just as important in ensuring that you are growing your networks and team of collaborators. This is true within your academic unit and the institution at large. Before we delve into hierarchies, let's first define what networking means.

The Oxford English Dictionary (n.d.-b) defines *networking* as "a system of trying to meet and talk to other people who may be useful to you in your work." Another definition of networking is "the action or process of interacting with others to exchange information and develop professional or social contacts" (Oxford English Dictionary, n.d.-b).

Based on these definitions, networking is not a haphazard form of meeting as many people as you can. Rather, it involves a system of meeting people—a system that is intentional and strategic. Most people cringe when they think about having to network, but it isn't as awful as it sounds. With a few basic principles, networking can be simpler than most people realize.

Determine the Purpose of Interactions

The first component of the networking definition deals with understanding the purpose of interactions and how the purpose will dictate the way you approach the networking situation. It is easy to abuse or misuse something when you do not understand its purpose. The same is true for networking. Understanding the purpose of the networking will also help manage your expectations related to the outcomes of the networking. Additionally, the purpose of the meeting or the networking experience might also determine the level of preparation needed prior to the meeting.

For example, networking to get to know a colleague across campus is different from networking with a potential collaborator on a grant proposal. This is true in terms of the mindset with which you approach the interaction, your expected outcomes, and the level of preparedness required for each type of meeting.

Let's say you are inviting some people to be coinvestigators on your grant proposal based on a very specific type of expertise they possess. Before you can even meet with the potential collaborator, you have to make sure you understand their program of research, their expertise, the specific role you want them to play on your team, and the time commitment required on their end. Also, you need to be able to explain your proposed research project well enough for them to understand why you need them on your team. Additionally, you will need to have an idea of how much time commitment will be required from them during the grant proposal development process. This information is necessary for the other people to gauge their interest, suitability, and availability to participate in your project. On the other hand, if you are meeting for coffee just to get to know someone better, some of the preparation addressed earlier may not be necessary.

Determine Which Connections Would Be Most Useful

The second component of the networking definition is related to the usefulness of the networking opportunity. What does *usefulness* mean? One might argue that any connection with people is useful for our daily life and well-being. However, for the purposes of professional networking, focus on connections that will be useful in your career progression. Connections are not all of equal importance. By adopting this mindset, you naturally start ranking your connections and ensuring that you are devoting the appropriate time and effort into the different relationships to make sure they flourish appropriately. This system provides a mental organization of your connections, which leads to a strategic prioritization of relationships based on their usefulness.

With every networking situation, ask yourself how useful this new connection is to you personally, professionally, or otherwise. It is great to know people just to know them; that is very important in our everyday lives, and all relationships must be valued. In fact, you never know what other connections may come from people you currently know. That is why you treat everyone with respect and dignity.

However, with professional networking, you have to adjust your perceptions related to the usefulness of a relationship so you can manage your expectations of what this individual can offer you or the connections they can help you make. Frustrations in networking and collaborations often stem from not understanding the usefulness of the relationship and therefore having extremely high and unrealistic expectations that cannot be met by an individual.

MERCY'S MOMENTS

I have had the great opportunity to be mentored by amazing human beings who have taken me under their wings and allowed me to grow. They have guided me and connected me with many notable scientists in my field, thereby growing my network and improving my chances of success as an early-career scientist.

A few years ago, in my quest to be mentored by diverse researchers with unique experiences, I was connected to a mentor who I thought would be a wonderful fit. She was driven, highly accomplished, and well-connected. She was great about answering my questions, pointing me in the right direction, and helping me find resources. However, at the time, I needed the most guidance on networking and growing my team of collaborators. It soon became very clear that she was willing to help me with everything as long as I did not ask her to provide a warm introduction to another person I needed to know professionally to reach my goals. This became a bone of contention for a while—I was frustrated, and she was frustrated too. One day, she mentioned in passing that when I asked her to introduce me to someone else to fill a gap in my career trajectory, it made her feel like she was not enough—and that I wanted other people to get the glory after she had helped me grow so much as a scientist.

Honestly, I understood her frustration. And maybe how I went about asking her to help me make connections was wrong. But no one person can be everything to you, and it is OK to ask for help from people other than your primary mentor in areas that you feel you are lacking. I was also quite uncomfortable with that conversation because sometimes mentors want to feel like they "made you." While there is some truth to this—mentors help you develop and grow as a professional by sharing their time, resources, and expertise—it is also true that you have made progress because you remained teachable and dedicated to your work, and you persevered through the difficult times. Yes, mentors make their protégés, but true mentors do not have to make their mentees feel like they owe them their lives at every corner. Through a series of events, I realized that I was expecting more from her than she was able to give me, and that was making both of us frustrated.

I had to quickly readjust my perception of the usefulness of this relationship to help me manage my expectations and avoid unnecessary frustrations. This did not mean she was a bad person; it just meant that there were some things I could not expect from her, and that was OK. It also taught me another important lesson about understanding the dynamics of relationships as you build your networks and collaborations. Some people are protectionists when it comes to networking, and you have to know how to navigate and manage those types of relationships. We delve into this in more detail later in this chapter.

Networking as an Exchange of Information

The second definition of networking brings out another very important concept—the exchange of information. Professional networking happens on a two-way street; a networking opportunity should benefit both individuals. We just talked about the usefulness of the networking, which is related to understanding the benefits you derive from the networking experience. However, never forget that what is true for you is also true for the other person. This begs an important question—what do you bring to the table?

Approaching networking as an exchange of information requires that you stay abreast with happenings in your chosen field or discipline. You have to be widely read; understand the evidence-based approaches, clinical guidelines, or other resources available in your field; and be familiar with leaders and stakeholders in your profession. You also need to know community stakeholders, regulatory bodies, and relevant policies and procedures governing your field or profession. Part of networking entails appropriately engaging in conversations on a myriad of topics and offering solutions. So, while I may not necessarily like listening to the news, I have to stay informed with what is happening in the world to remain relevant.

Take Inventory of Your Strengths

So, what do you bring to the table? Taking inventory of your skills, knowledge, gifts, and talents is a task many of us do not do naturally. We are often told that we are being prideful when we emphasize our strengths. But being humble does not mean that you deny the ways in which you are skilled, knowledgeable, gifted, or talented. You can acknowledge your own strengths while also respecting the fact that other people may be uniquely skilled, knowledgeable, talented, or gifted in other ways. There is room for all of us to grow and be successful without being condescending to others or belittling their efforts. As such, successful people understand their strengths and have learned the art of leveraging their strengths to produce more successes, and you should do the same.

You might say this is easier said than done. Where and how do I get started with evaluating what I bring to the table?

Start by asking yourself these important questions:

- What strengths do I bring to the networking table?
- When am I most effective?
- In what types of environments do I thrive?
- How can I add value to someone else?
- How can I create opportunities for others?

SWOT Analysis

Another strategy to evaluate what you bring to the table is to conduct a SWOT analysis. A SWOT analysis is a tool you can utilize to take inventory of your skills, knowledge, gifts, and talents (Teoli et al., 2021). SWOT stands for strengths, weaknesses, opportunities, and threats. In its broader context, it is used for organizations or groups, but I often encourage individuals to conduct a critical analysis of their own strengths, weaknesses, opportunities, and threats. Understanding these important concepts makes you aware of not only what types of individuals you need to cover your weak areas but also what you bring to the networking table as a professional.

Conducting a personal SWOT analysis will further guide you toward what types of networking opportunities you should pursue. For example, if you find that one of your weaknesses is research methodology but you are developing a research project that requires the use of a specific research methodology, approaching another researcher who has extensive experience in this area may prove very useful.

Having a good understanding of what you bring to the table will help prevent you from unintentionally getting into situations that set you up for failure because you approached the wrong person. If you understand this concept, you will limit your professional networking and collaborations to those interactions that have the potential to yield the desired results. Additionally, when you complete a SWOT analysis, you will learn to appropriately gauge the value you bring to the table by completing a critical analysis of your expertise. This will prevent you from overselling or underselling your expertise, both of which are potentially detrimental to your career. You don't want to oversell yourself because then you run the risk of overcommitting and underdelivering. You also don't want to undersell yourself because you may miss out on opportunities where you are inadvertently deemed underqualified.

Thus, outside understanding the value you bring to the table, completing the SWOT analysis will ultimately save you time and resources by ensuring that you only engage with opportunities that are appropriate for you and your stage of career development. Ultimately, this limits the potential for frustration. As you already know, time is a very important commodity in academia.

Conducting a SWOT analysis will also help you identify your strengths and opportunities so you can market yourself in a favorable light. This makes people view you as a resource, an expert, and someone they would like on their team to increase their own value. The secret in applying the SWOT analysis lies in identifying the various ways in which you could add value to the people you meet as you build relationships and connections. We will cover this concept in greater detail in Chapters 5 and 6.

Using the chart provided, list (in order of importance) four strengths, weaknesses, opportunities, and threats. After you are done, ask yourself what types of connections will help you fill areas of need so that you can set yourself up for success.

Strengths	Weaknesses	Opportunities	Threats
1.	1.	1.	1.
2.	2.	2.	2.
3.	3.	3.	3.
4.	4.	4.	4.

SUCCESS NUGGET

Do not network aimlessly. First define the purpose of the networking, then determine its usefulness. Make sure the networking is a mutually beneficial situation by adding value to the relationship through the exchange of information. Remember, all connections are not created equal, and you should be intentional with understanding your strengths, weaknesses, opportunities, and threats and how they might impact the networking encounter.

Strategies for Creating Meaningful Networks and Collaborations

Now that you know what type of people you need on your team to help fill gaps in your expertise, it is important to learn some strategies to create meaningful collaborations and grow your network in academia.

Practice Building Trust

Academia tends to have a reputation of sabotage and obstructions, thus stymieing collaborations and networking opportunities.

One strategy for creating meaningful relationships is to establish yourself as a trustworthy, dependable, and loyal individual. These are necessary soft skills in the workplace and are paramount to the development and maintenance of strategic relationships. We will delve into each of these attributes separately, but I want to underscore the fact that people are more likely to collaborate with you if you possess these qualities.

According to Ken Blanchard (2014), seven ways to be dependable are:

- Delivering on your promises
- Being timely
- Being responsive
- Being organized
- Being accountable
- Being consistent
- Following up on assignments and projects

If you say you are going to do something, do it and make sure you meet expectations related to the quantity and quality of the work done. Additionally, complete the work by the stipulated deadline. If you are not able to deliver by the agreed-upon deadline, communicate in a timely manner, and offer an alternative completion date. Life happens and we all know that, but communication is key. Similarly, your responsiveness is an indicator of the value you assign to the network or individual. Therefore, the speed with which you respond to people can be an indicator of how much you value the relationship. Make sure you are sending the right signals to the people in your network.

Furthermore, being organized and accountable for your work can increase other people's perceptions of your dependability because possessing these qualities increases perceptions of ability to complete tasks. Following up on assignments or projects indicates that you have a vested interest in the success of the project. I recommend that you follow up with people in your network when you know they are working on something that is important to them, even if the project doesn't directly benefit you. This shows that you are interested in other people's success. Lastly, being consistent is crucial. It is not enough to practice these values sometimes. They must become consistent practices.

> *"Success does not come from what you do occasionally, it comes from what you do consistently."*
>
> *–Marie Forleo*

In addition to this list, I believe other ways you can increase your dependability, trustworthiness, and loyalty include:

- Offering to help others when appropriate
- Sharing information as necessary
- Safeguarding information shared with you in confidence

If you consistently do this, people begin to view you as someone they can trust and depend on—and who will be loyal to them and protect their interests.

Identify the Needs of Others

The second strategy for building meaningful collaborations is developing a keen interest in the needs of others and offering to be part of the solution. Paying attention to details as you naturally interact with people will help you identity their needs, even if they don't explicitly share them. When people feel that they are valued, their experiences are validated, and their concerns are heard, they gravitate toward you and allow themselves to be vulnerable. People often do not want to admit that they are struggling or needing help. Developing empathy and an ability to decipher what people need without their telling you is an invaluable asset and soft skill in helping you build meaningful and long-lasting collaborations and relationships.

Offer Solutions

Identifying other people's needs is an important skill to possess; however, what will solidify the relationship even further is your ability to offer solutions to identified problems or needs. Even if you do not have the solution, your willingness to brainstorm, offer suggestions, and provide connections to others who might have the answers will help you form a more meaningful relationship with people. I highly encourage you to be genuinely thoughtful and caring when doing this. People can recognize pretentious efforts, and that does the opposite of building trustworthiness, dependability, and loyalty. Remember, when people feel that you are genuinely interested in them as human beings and they are not just a connection on your contact list, they will likely look out for your interests and reciprocate your kind gestures.

Share Your Strengths With Others

The next strategy to build meaningful collaborations is to genuinely work on adding value, not merely selling yourself. What do I mean by this? Some people tend to advertise how skilled they are at something but never add value to others based on their strengths. For example, if someone is good with technology but refuses to share their knowledge with others, they may be labeled as an individual who wants others to be at their mercy—they want people who need help in that particular area to seek them out as the only expert around.

What people forget sometimes is that when you are the only one who can do something in your organization or college, then all requests will come to you. If doing this particular task is part of your job description, then that is absolutely fine. However, if this is something you are doing only when you are able to, then you run the risk of overcommitting by saying yes to everyone or seeming unhelpful when you can't say yes to everyone. Therefore, sharing your strengths and training others can in fact help you to be productive too by investing time in other areas of your life. Be generous with your strengths.

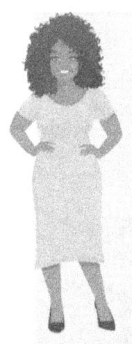

MERCY'S MOMENTS

Grant writing is one of the skills I have developed over the last several years as an early-career scientist. I have been quite successful in securing grant funding from various sources, and I often get questions from people on how to develop competitive grant proposals. Last year, I thought I would actually help more people by developing a seminar series on grant writing for early-career scientists that focused on the National Institutes of Health grant application process. The seminar series had four parts and was well received.

When I first developed this idea, I thought that I was only going to present the information to early science investigators at my university. But through my networks, the registration flyer was widely shared with people from all over the world on various social media platforms. What started as a small project aimed at sharing some strategies on developing competitive grant proposals soon snowballed into a global event with over 100 attendees from the United States, Europe, Africa, and Asia. My willingness to share my strengths led me to build additional networks across the globe and continued to solidify my reputation as a developing scientist. What I learned from this experience is that when we willingly share our strengths and talents, the universe has a way of giving back to us in even greater ways than we would have anticipated.

Acknowledge Your Weaknesses

The opposite scenario to what is described above may also be true. You may need help with something, and your coworker is knowledgeable in that area. Instead of humbly asking for help, you try to do it yourself because you don't want to feel inferior. Remember when we talked about SWOT? The "W" stands for weaknesses. Yes, we all have them. We can also call them areas of opportunity, but the honest truth is that we cannot be good at everything, and we need other people. Building meaningful relationships requires us to safely disclose our weaknesses to others so they can help us.

Notice I said *safely*. We should not disclose our weaknesses to every person we encounter because some people will use them against us. Unfortunately, that's just how the world works sometimes, and it happens in academia quite often. A friend of mine likes to say that not everyone should be in your business. And she is right. People should earn your trust before you can safely disclose your weaknesses to them.

If we are willing to safely admit when we need help from others and allow them to share their expertise with us, they can relate to us as human beings. Ultimately, this helps us build meaningful relationships because, frankly, no one likes a know-it-all. This strategy has helped me grow as a professional and scientist. I'm not afraid to acknowledge my weaknesses and to ask for help. If you have a teachable attitude, other people will share their strengths with you, which makes them feel that they are adding value to their relationship with you. It humanizes you and allows other people to positively contribute to your growth and development in a meaningful way.

Choose Your Alliances Carefully

Another important strategy is to align yourself with the right people. Earlier in this chapter, I talked about formal and informal hierarchies in academia. While formal hierarchies are important in opening doors for you, it's important to decipher informal hierarchies because they often provide networking opportunities that may lead to personal and professional successes.

Informal hierarchies can be either positive or negative, depending on the agenda and outcome being propagated. These hierarchies are often perpetuated by unspoken rules that if not understood, may destroy you. I would like for all informal hierarchies to be positive, but this is not always the case in academia. It is imperative that you differentiate between the negative and positive as soon as possible.

Informal leaders and influencers in your college or institution may hold the keys to progression in a certain area. Know who they are, but more importantly, find out whom they can influence within your college or institution. This is equally important whether the informal hierarchy is positive or negative. I want to emphasize that you should have cordial and professional working relationships with all your colleagues. But, depending on what your objectives are, make sure to align yourself with the right individuals or groups.

> **MATCHING ALLIANCES WITH PROFESSIONAL GOALS**
>
> Let's say that your objective is to be a nationally recognized clinical expert in gerontological nursing. It would be important to align yourself with individuals who have national connections to professionals and opportunities in this area. You should be most concerned about building meaningful and mutually beneficial relationships with individuals who share your values and are most likely to help launch your career into your desired trajectory. Therefore, the critical questions to ask are: What is your desired outcome for the alignment? Is this alignment

congruent with your personal values and beliefs? And what is the opportunity cost of aligning yourself with a certain individual or group? This brings us back to the two important components of networking—purpose and usefulness.

One of the things people do not usually consider is that there is often opportunity cost associated with any alignment in your networking endeavors. The Oxford English Dictionary (n.d.-c) defines *opportunity cost* as "the loss of potential gain from other alternatives when one alternative is chosen." Whether you like it or not, in most cases, by choosing to align yourself with a particular individual or group, there are certain opportunities, resources, or other networks that might be outside of your grasp. Therefore, making sure that you understand the opportunity cost of the alignment will help you make informed decisions about which networks to belong to.

Another way to strategically align your alliances with your professional goals is to volunteer for specific causes. Volunteering strategically can help you build skills, grow your network in a particular field, and create meaningful collaborations while serving your community through your expertise. Opportunities can be as simple as volunteering for a professional conference or for a task force created to solve a problem at the college. Being selective when choosing volunteer opportunities ensures mutual benefit. We delve more into this concept in Chapter 4.

Social Media as a Networking Tool

Finally, consider how you can use social media effectively to grow your network and create meaningful relationships that are outside of your day-to-day significant relationships. This area is receiving increased attention from the professional world. About a decade ago, it was almost frowned upon for professionals to use social media platforms to promote their work. The tide has certainly changed. I was surprised about two years ago when a scientific journal accepted my manuscript for publication and staff asked for my social media handles so they could promote their journal and highlight my work by tagging me on my various social media profiles. In that moment, it became clear to me that professional propagation on social media is here to stay. It can be a useful tool in growing your network, building collaborations, and increasing the impact of your work if done well.

The evolution of social media for professional use has also led to the proliferation of social media platforms that are specifically targeted toward promoting professional identity, growing professional networks, and expanding the impact and reach of one's work. You can even use social media to learn about new job opportunities in your industry. Social media can also be a valuable tool to discover new ideas and trends as well as building and enhancing your professional brand (Sreenivasan, 2017).

Understanding the "voice" to use on various platforms is also very important. For example, how you relay information on Twitter, LinkedIn, or Facebook might be different because you are communicating with different audiences. See below for an illustration.

- Facebook: OMG!!! I'm so excited to share that I just won the early-career investigator award from XXX. I really worked so hard the last few years to earn this recognition. I want to thank all my family and friends who have consistently supported me and believed in me as well as my colleague XXX for nominating me.

- Twitter: Thank you to XXX for selecting me as their 2021 recipient of the early-career investigator award. I'm honored by this gesture. Thank you to Dr. XXX for nominating me for this award.

- LinkedIn: I'm greatly honored to share that I have won the 2021 early-career investigator award from XXX. XXX is the leading research society for addictions scientists. I would like to thank my colleague, Dr. XXX, who nominated me for this award.

With the advent of using social media platforms for professional reasons, there are misses and hits, and one should be aware of the dos and don'ts of social media use for professional reasons. From an article by Gerri Detweiler (2018) that compiles advice from 10 experts in the field, below are some tips that might be helpful in advancing your career or business by using your social media presence wisely:

- Lead with objectives: Know the objective for posting on social media, who your target audience is, and the message you are trying to convey.

- Build with authority: Establish why you are the right person to convey this message. Emphasize your expertise and training in a particular field, and grow your authority base by increasing credibility.

- Start a timely conversation: This means that you have to keep up with what is trending in your field or industry to ensure you are appropriately engaging your audiences.

- Show appreciation for others: Acknowledge other people's contributions and success. Share important causes on your platforms so that you can also highlight other people's work. This will grow your networks and build comradery.

- Stand out and create a niche: Create a niche for your social media presence and a persona that will consistently promote your personal brand. There are millions of people on social medial platforms; therefore, you need to give people a reason to follow you.

- Have a clear goal: Social media can be used for many reasons. You have to be sure you understand why you are using social media. Outside of professional networking and brand building, social media can offer opportunities to monetize your brand, if that is something you are interested in.

- Dominate on one platform: Although it is advisable to keep up with as many social media platforms as possible, pick one or two that will be your primary platform(s). This is important in ensuring that your efforts are consistent, and your target audience remains clear.

- Plan your social media activity: Believe it or not, growing your professional brand on social media requires strategic and intentional activity. Do not post just for the sake of posting. Determine how often you can realistically update your audiences, and remain consistent in your messaging.

- Use appropriate visual aids when possible: People are more likely to engage with your content if it is visually appealing. Make sure that visual aids are appropriate for your audiences.

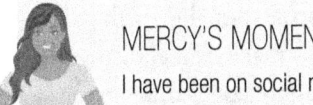

MERCY'S MOMENTS

I have been on social media for many years. Like most people, I initially used social media only for personal and social connections. I didn't use these platforms for professional reasons until I started working on my PhD. As I continued to grow professionally, I noticed a trend toward creating an online professional identity. In the past, we only read textbooks, books, autobiographies, or published scientific work of successful people, but times have changed. Nowadays, it is not enough to be an expert that only scholars know about. You have to promote your work and yourself to consistently add value for people who follow your work.

When I started using social media professionally, my goal was not to be a Hollywood influencer but rather to slowly build my brand as a nurse scientist who would eventually be respected as an expert in my field. I was intentional in building my professional presence online, and I have gained many connections and opportunities through social media engagement.

My current position is one of those opportunities. My dean found me on LinkedIn and invited me to interview at our college. I had never thought about moving to Alabama to pursue a career as a tenure-track assistant professor. Although this was not what I had planned, it was the best career decision I have made so far. This opportunity would not have been possible if I had not actively promoted myself and my work online.

> **SUCCESS NUGGET**
>
> To create meaningful collaborations and grow your network in academia, establish yourself as trustworthy and dependable, show a keen interest in the needs of others and provide solutions, add value to each relationship, ask for help in areas where you are weak, align yourself with the right people, and use social media to promote your professional identity and brand.

Strategic Classifications of Networks and Collaborations

It feels odd to say that collaborations and networks have classifications. This is because we know that we need to treat all people with dignity and respect, regardless of whether we think they have the potential to contribute to our personal or professional growth. Classifying our contacts and networks might also make us feel disingenuous or insincere. However, if you do not classify your connections and relationships appropriately, you could set yourself up for failure because you will not invest the appropriate energies and resources to your most important connections.

A famous televangelist, Bishop T. D. Jakes (2016), posits that three types of people play roles in our lives: confidants, constituents, and comrades. It is important to properly classify which people in your life belong to each of these categories.

Confidants

Confidants support you and are interested in helping you develop as a person. They are neither afraid of you showing weaknesses and frailty nor intimidated by your strengths or successes. These are people you can trust with your life. They celebrate and uphold you, and they cover your weaknesses when necessary to protect you from those who may not have your best interests at heart. Confidants can strategically catapult you personally or professionally and have a wide network of influential people they are eager to connect you with. They will be in your life for a very long time. Cultivating these relationships continually will be vital for your long-term success and growth. Therefore, find meaningful ways to also add value to their lives.

Constituents

Constituents possess values similar to yours. They are in your life because they support what you stand for. Constituents are important because they help you actualize your vision and are willing to connect you with their networks to ensure your success. They may not be in your life for extended periods, and you may not consistently work with them. However, if you need someone to carry your vision, you can call on them and they will be available. They will invest time and resources in you for a limited period.

Comrades

Comrades, on the other hand, are against what you are against. They may not agree with you about everything, but they are willing to collaborate to defeat a common enemy or solve a common problem. It sounds crude, but comrades are equally important to you. They may be beneficial for covering your blind spots. They protect you from others they believe are unfair to you—or even people who may want to destroy you—but what they attack is also beneficial for them. So, it's not really about you. They have a vested interest in you succeeding at a particular task or issue because your win is their win too.

Comrades are not your regular, everyday pal. Once you have conquered the common enemy or resolved the issue, the collaboration will dissipate or dissolve. It is important to understand the temporary nature of this relationship because it may need to be terminated or reclassified. Holding onto this relationship past its expiration date or failing to reclassify the relationship's purpose or usefulness might hurt you in the long run.

Power Connectors

Another way to categorize connections is by what Judy Robinett (2014) calls *power connectors*. These high-level connections in your network act as bridges between you and other networks or between two or more well-established networks. They maintain influence across various spheres. Through them, you can gain access to a strategically interwoven network that has more resources, thereby providing more impact for your work.

Power connectors are often generous and set the example of adding value to the network without expecting anything in return. The more power connectors you establish relationships with, the more exponential benefits you can reap from their networks. Power connectors have a reputation for connecting the best people with the best resources, and they enjoy linking eager and enthusiastic people. As you work on growing your networks and collaborations in academia, be sure to identify the power connectors in your college or institution. It will serve your career progression well.

> **SUCCESS NUGGET**
>
> In her book *Your Network Is Your Net Worth,* Porter Gale (2013) explores strategies to unlock the power of connections. As we build collaborations, the synergistic value, goodwill, resources, and connections that are formed have the potential to unlock hidden doors that only people in the network have access to, the ability to learn about opportunities that others only dream about, and the expertise to draw from to make your collective expertise valuable. Your network is your currency in academia—use it wisely.

> ## TOP 5, KEY 50, VITAL 100
>
> In academia, as in life, your network is important in unlocking doors that others may not even know exist, which allows you to achieve success more quickly. Understanding the importance of networking and collaboration ensures that you nurture the appropriate connections. Because you have limited time and resources, maximizing your networks requires a strategic evaluation of your connections and relationships to help you determine where to invest the most time and resources and which relationships you need to continue adding value to.
>
> To achieve this, I suggest that you follow the 5 + 50 +100 power circles rule by Judy Robinett (2014). She emphasizes the importance of evaluating your network and relationships and appropriately classifying them into these three categories: your top 5, your key 50, and your vital 100 connections and relationships.
>
> Top 5
>
> Your top 5 relationships are people you connect with nearly every day. They are your closest friends, family, or business associates. They likely would qualify as confidants, as we discussed earlier. You can trust these people with your life and should therefore be intentional in continually adding value to the relationships.
>
> Key 50
>
> Your key 50 relationships are significant to your growth and success because they add value to your life and professional career. You should connect with these people regularly and nurture the relationships.
>
> Vital 100
>
> The last category is your vital 100 people. You stay in contact with your vital 100 at least once a month. You can call on them when needed, and you continue to add value to them.

Final Thoughts

The quality of your connections and networks is more important than the quantity. After all, networking should be a strategic system of meeting people and maintaining relationships that are useful for your growth and development as a person or professional. In this chapter, we have explored the secrets of networking that if successfully implemented can lead to exponential growth and success in your chosen field. Happy networking!

4

SERVICE AND ACADEMIC CITIZENSHIP

Welcome to Chapter 4. I call this the fun chapter because in most cases, people volunteer for causes they are passionate about or in areas where they want to make a difference. Therefore, in that sense, service can and should be a fun aspect of your life. This is the part of your academic role where you have the most autonomy (except for the required service expectations for your college), which also contributes to the fun aspect of service. My genuine hope is that people are serving because they have a vested interest in the opportunity and want to see positive outcomes. I'm not oblivious to the fact that this is not always the case, and we discuss that later in the chapter. But first things first.

In this chapter, we explore the meaning of service and academic citizenship, their value in academia, the types of service opportunities available, and ways to balance service with the other parts of your educator role. I should warn you from the start that service can be fun and very fulfilling, but it can easily lead to overcommitment and become a nightmare in what seems like a blink of an eye. That is why we will also talk about how to prioritize service, when to know that you are overcommitted, and what implications service and academic citizenship have for your personal and professional life.

What Is Academic Citizenship?

As you already know from Chapter 1, service and academic citizenship are important components of your academic role. For the purpose of this book, we will use service and academic citizenship interchangeably.

I like the definition of *academic citizenship* offered by University of York (n.d., para. 1–2), which states:

> Academic citizenship covers activities additional to 'normal' teaching and research. It encompasses a broad range of externally and internally focused contributions and is defined as engagement with those elements of university life that enable the smooth and collegial operation of the institution.

Miami University (n.d., para. 7) defines *service* this way:

> Service applies a faculty member's knowledge, skills, and expertise as an educator, a member of a discipline or profession, or a participant in an institution to benefit students, the institution, the discipline or profession, and the community in a manner consistent with the missions of the university and the campus.

As you can see from the definitions, academic citizenship can be a vague concept and often is misunderstood. This is why you should first know how service and academic citizenship are defined and evaluated within your academic unit or the institution by familiarizing yourself with the policies and procedures governing this important component of your role. While it is commendable to serve in various roles, you should be aware of which activities count within your department, and make sure that you are participating in opportunities that enrich you not only personally but also professionally.

Note that the Miami University definition references applying your knowledge, skills, and expertise. I hope that as you choose service opportunities, you will be guided by this principle. Also, remember that although you will benefit from service opportunities, the ultimate and true goal of service is to enrich your students, your institution, your profession, and your community.

There are several opportunities for service and academic citizenship, and they can be categorized as follows:

- Service at the college level
- Service to the university
- Service to professional organizations
- Service to the community

Service at the College Level

Let's start with exploring service at the college level. Normally, you will have two types of service opportunities: mandatory and optional. For example, most colleges or academic units have standing committees to which faculty are either assigned or elected. These committees have a specific function and purpose and are designed to help the academic unit operate smoothly.

By virtue of being a faculty member, you are required to attend certain faculty organization meetings. If you have a valid reason to miss, you must obtain prior approval. In my case, because I teach both undergraduate and graduate students, I am also expected to attend the undergraduate faculty and graduate faculty committee meetings.

In addition to these general committees, I might be assigned to another specific committee—for example, the Student Life Committee, whose purpose is to determine and address the needs, expectations, and preferences of students by employing meaningful strategies to build relationships, thus promoting students' satisfaction with the college or academic unit. I may also have mandatory advising requirements for students and mentoring of junior faculty. What I have described may be similar to or different from your requirements. Therefore, it is important to learn what the minimum required service is for your college.

Knowing this will allow you to plan for your other service opportunities, both within and outside the college. Notice that up to this point, we have talked only about the required service opportunities. We haven't even addressed the other opportunities you might be interested in and would love to contribute to. That is why voluntary opportunities for service are also available. For example, because I'm passionate about research and scholarly productivity, I also choose to serve on the Scholarly Affairs Committee, a voluntary committee that addresses scholarship needs of faculty within the college. In addition, I volunteer as a faculty advisor in the undergraduate peer-mentoring program and occasionally for a task force convened to address a particular issue in our college.

In Chapter 3, I addressed the significant concept of diversifying your network. Choosing your service opportunities wisely can also help you enrich your network both within and outside your academic unit or college. While your college will appreciate your volunteer work, leave room for other opportunities that may arise outside your college—and be flexible enough to jump on those opportunities as they become available.

MERCY'S MOMENTS

A couple of years ago, I volunteered to work on a task force to restructure how some of our second-semester courses are offered. Our traditional bachelor of science in nursing (BSN) is a five-semester program. We traditionally admitted students to the program only in the summer and fall. The college was expanding enrollment by adding an additional admission semester in the spring.

This meant that we would have students completing their second semester courses in the summer, including the Fundamentals of Professional Nursing, a clinical course. This was the first time we would offer a clinical course requiring 180 clinical hours in a limited summer term. Our task force was tasked with (no pun intended) figuring out how to restructure this course while ensuring that student learning outcomes were met. Completing all the work related to this task force required several planning and brainstorming meetings with other members of the task force and administrators. We also had to work on updating course documents to reflect the new course structure.

As you can see, with just a few mandatory committees and only three volunteer opportunities, my plate is getting full, which limits what else I can do outside the college. Although these volunteer opportunities might be fun and rewarding, they can quickly fill up your days without you realizing it. And remember, this is only one aspect of your job.

SUCCESS NUGGET

Being cognizant that there is more to your academic role than service will keep your mind open to opportunities outside your academic unit, which may help you grow in other areas and expose you to different networks—thereby growing your influence and impact.

Service to the University

Don't forget to ask about service opportunities outside your academic unit and how you can participate based on your areas of expertise. The caveat for university service is that I usually recommend that you first get comfortable serving within your academic unit and understand its strategic plan, organization structure, operations, and priorities before you seek out university service opportunities. This is because most of the time, when you serve on a university committee, you are representing the interests of your academic unit or college. By default, you are your college's ambassador. You cannot be a worthy ambassador when you do not understand your own academic unit's operations and priorities. In my opinion, this is dangerous and a sure way to grossly misrepresent the interests of your college. This is not the time for "fake it till you make it."

Some university opportunities are elected service positions, some are volunteer, and others are appointed. If you are going to pursue this type of service, I highly recommend that you first speak with your supervisor or dean to determine whether other opportunities will better fit your interests and expertise. Ensuring that you have the support of your college will make you more confident and increase your effectiveness in your new university service position, especially if it is a volunteer opportunity. Furthermore, it is important to understand that with university service, there is an expectation that you will report back to your academic unit or college to ensure dissemination and understanding of information conveyed from the university level to the college level.

LEADERSHIP IS NOT A RACE

Another important consideration when it comes to service opportunities is whether you are serving as a committee member or holding a leadership position, such as chair or vice chair of the committee. Some committees (both at the college and university level) may have specific requirements, such as tenure and experience, for serving as chair or vice chair, while others may not. The level of engagement and time commitment will obviously be different for a committee member than a chair or vice chair. I recommend that you weigh not only the pros and cons of each type of committee membership but also how it is viewed within your college for evaluation purposes. Obviously, all service is appreciated and encouraged, but serving as chair of a committee carries more weight than simply being a member.

At any rate, avoid overcommitment; for example, you shouldn't be chairing three different committees when you are first starting out, in addition to managing your teaching and other important aspects of your job. I have seen junior faculty who have taken on more service leadership opportunities than they have time for and have ended up sacrificing their mental health and losing work-life balance because they are overcommitted. I personally recommend that you refrain from service leadership positions when you are new to your academic role, unless it is a requirement—for example, if you were hired into a specific administrative role that requires you to chair a particular committee.

This may sound counterintuitive. You should be diving into every opportunity to show that you are committed to your new role and your new home, right? Wrong! Stepping into service leadership positions you are not adequately prepared to take on actually sets you up for failure, decreases your confidence, increases your anxiety, and affects your productivity in other areas of your job. It also has the potential to disrupt your work-life balance, especially if there are overcommitment issues as well. We will delve more into this topic in Chapter 9.

Part of my reasoning for this recommendation is that you are still learning about your organization's policies and procedures and other relevant operational complexities. Think about it this way: You wouldn't want your new graduate nurse who is still in orientation to be suddenly thrust into the charge nurse role.

Unfortunately, this sometimes happens where there are severe shortages of nurses, but it still does not represent a safe clinical situation. This is the same for service leadership positions. There are some instances when you can volunteer to help when there isn't anyone more experienced to step into the role, but this should be for a limited time frame.

Let me emphasize that this recommendation is not based on perceptions of lack of ability or suitability for the leadership role. In my experience, people new to their positions or the organization often have great ideas on how to solve problems, improve processes, and optimize outcomes, and they may have experience that would make them good candidates for service leadership positions. I also encourage people to take on leadership positions that are appropriate for their career trajectory as well as current professional status and do not inadvertently stymie their potential and productivity in other important areas. Therefore, exercising wisdom on when to take on leadership roles is important. Moreover, as a new faculty member, you should still significantly contribute to the success of your committee, whether you are a committee member or the chair of the committee.

Here's my rationale: Serving as a member before taking the lead allows you the opportunity to understand the dynamics and mission of the group—and it also teaches you to be a team player first. Why is this important? In Chapter 3, we discussed that one way to create meaningful and strategic relationships is to support others and help them be successful, without expecting the gesture to be reciprocated. When you genuinely show kindness and concern, people gravitate toward you.

When you support people when they are in leadership positions and you help them meet their goals, objectives, and targets, you show that you are invested in the success of the team, not just you as an individual. Eventually you will establish yourself as a dependable team player who supports others. In turn, your colleagues will be willing to support you in future leadership endeavors. And honestly, you might be viewed as overzealous if you are taking on too many leadership roles when you first start your position. So, take your time before jumping into a leadership role—it's not a race.

Service to Professional Organizations

Another important type is service to a professional organization. Professional service can be local, regional, national, or international. Similar to service in academia, these opportunities may be elected, appointed, or strictly voluntary. Elected positions are considered prestigious and may provide more perks during annual merit evaluations. Some appointed positions are also considered prestigious, depending on who is doing the appointment and the organization, committee, or task force to which someone is appointed. Volunteer positions, which are often based on interests and expertise in a specific area, provide additional opportunities for service. Depending on your previous level of professional organization involvement (prior to assuming your academic role), all of these levels of professional organization engagement and service may be appropriate as you transition to academia.

For example, if you are an advanced practice registered nurse and have been serving for a few years on your state board of nursing task force for implementing full practice authority, it may be appropriate to consider a national-level service opportunity. This service can be elected, appointed, or strictly on a volunteer basis—even though you are new to your academic role.

With professional service, I often tell people to gauge what the next appropriate level of service is based on previous experience. It would not make sense for you to pursue an international-level service opportunity when you do not have any experience serving at the local, regional, or national level in that particular area. You can also use a tiered approach whereby you try to maintain relevance at each level, as long as you do not take on too many service obligations.

The same argument that was true with college- and university-level service is true for professional organization service; time commitments will vary significantly between being a committee member and chairing a committee—let alone leading an entire organization. Therefore, while professional service is highly encouraged, take an honest inventory of your time, resources, and expertise to ensure that you can provide valuable service to the professional organization you choose. I sometimes run into people who acquire service positions with professional organizations like they are badges of honor to be displayed. This is not only the wrong approach but also detrimental to service.

Make sure that when you commit, you have the time, expertise, and passion to appropriately contribute. If this is not the case, professional organizations may run on the backs of only a few individuals, which negatively affects those who are doing all the work to ensure the organization runs smoothly. This is simply unprofessional; people will see that you are not dependable and do not care about the success of the organization. And by the way, we live in a small world, and news travels fast; you may think that no one is noticing or sharing their experiences of working with you, but in the long run, people will not recommend you for other opportunities because you are unreliable.

One time, I was talking with some people about a service opportunity that was available through a professional organization. Several names were tossed out as potential candidates. It was quite interesting to me that when one name was suggested, several people noted that this person was quick to say yes to service opportunities but didn't follow through. That is when it clicked for me. Professional service opportunities are not simply boxes to check. A "been there, done that" attitude will not take you far in the world of professional service. People notice, and your reputation—whether good or bad—will precede you, which can have professional ramifications. Therefore, as you seek professional service opportunities, regardless of whether they are in local, state, regional, national, or international spheres, only commit to opportunities when you have the time, enthusiasm, resources, expertise, and dedication to serve. People will respect you more if you say no for a good reason than if you always say yes but underdeliver.

> **SUCCESS NUGGET**
>
> Professional service opportunities are not simply boxes to check. A "been there, done that" attitude will not take you far in the world of professional service and networking; people notice, and your reputation—whether good or bad—will precede you. As much as depends on you, make sure when people say, "I've heard a lot about you," it's for good reasons.

MERCY'S MOMENTS

While I highly recommend that you join professional organizations and serve in various capacities, I want to caution you against joining too many organizations. Yes, there is such a thing. As an enthusiastic, newly graduated tenure-track assistant professor, I found myself trapped in a cycle of professional organization membership renewals. I naively thought that the more professional organizations I joined, the more member benefits I would enjoy, and perhaps I would have more outlets for disseminating my research. Over the years, I learned that for the most part, professional organizations offer similar membership packages and perks. What differentiates them are the scope and mission of the organizations, the target audience, and the diversity of opportunities available to members.

One day, I received the infamous email reminder that my membership to a professional organization was expiring in 30 days. As I got my wallet to start working on renewal, it dawned on me that I belonged to three organizations with similar missions, target audiences, and programming. The fact that membership dues had significantly increased for many of the organizations I belonged to precipitated my thoughtful reevaluation. Paying three annual subscriptions to receive similar benefits was not cost-effective, and there was no additional value in belonging to all three organizations. I quickly sat down and thoroughly examined my professional organization memberships to make sure that I was not only maximizing what I got for my money but also diversifying my experiences and networks to promote true professional growth.

It Takes More Than Just Being a Member

Your role as a member of an organization should not end with paying your membership dues and perhaps attending the national conference. I recommend active engagement in many aspects of your organization's programming and governance. This approach will be important for growing your expertise, expanding your network, and influencing policy at various levels. Therefore, it's not the quantity of the organizations that matters; it's the diversity of the experiences you receive from your memberships, the opportunities to participate in organizational governance, and the richness of the networks available to you through your memberships.

My advice is to be systematic and strategic with your professional organization memberships. Aim to have at least one international or national membership to a nonspecialty organization, such as Sigma Theta Tau International or the National League for Nursing. Then join at least one regional research society (especially if research and scholarship are major components of your job description), such as the Southern Nursing Research Society or the Midwest Nursing Research Society. Also become a member of one specialty-specific organization, such as the American Association for Critical-Care Nurses, and participate in your local state nurses association.

Finally, I recommend that you belong to at least one organization that is interdisciplinary but champions a particular area of interest. In my case, this is the College of Drug Dependence and Problems and the Society for Behavioral Medicine. A multidisciplinary organization introduces another level of professional networking that may not otherwise be available to you if you just stay within your nursing circles, thereby promoting interprofessional collaboration.

> **SUCCESS NUGGET**
>
> What truly matters with professional organization memberships is the diversity of the experiences you receive, the opportunities to participate in organizational governance at various levels, and the richness of the networks available to you through your memberships. The quality of membership perks derived from your professional memberships should supersede the quantity of professional memberships.

Service to the Community

Community service includes activities that you engage in to serve your community. It may or may not be directly related to your professional career objectives. For example, you could serve on your daughter's local school board or deliver free food to people in need. Community service may also include working with your local religious organization to provide free clothes to people at the local homeless shelter. As with the other types of service, it is important to determine how much time you have to commit to community service activities.

Notably, many universities and other institutions of higher learning are now paying more attention to community service, resulting in a rise in philanthropic activities that are spearheaded by the universities. It is, therefore, a great time to couple your academic citizenship with other philanthropic work that is championed by your institution. This allows you to pursue service opportunities you are truly passionate about while supporting the mission of your institution.

Paid Versus Unpaid Service Opportunities

When you are in academia, carefully consider the roles you engage with, especially those outside the university. You should familiarize yourself with your university's policies and procedures related to outside work that is compensated. You need to know what has to be reported, the reporting period, and the frequency of reporting. You also must appropriately disclose any potential and actual conflicts of interest that may arise because of your paid or unpaid service positions.

When not handled correctly, this situation could potentially land you in legal trouble. When in doubt, always run the issue by your dean, supervisors, or whoever is responsible as stipulated in the policy. It is better to be safe than sorry. Conflicts of interest are not inherently bad as long as they are disclosed appropriately. This is especially important in an academic environment. Your university wants to know that outside activities will not place you under undue influence that may jeopardize the interests and security of the organization. With due diligence, you have nothing to worry about.

All four types of service opportunities we have discussed have their place. Depending on the stage of your career, one type of service may be more important to your progression as an academic than another; however, never neglect to engage in service opportunities related to causes you love. Serve simply because you want to, not because it counts on your evaluation. When you are in an academic environment, it is very easy to lose the passion and the why behind what you do. The most rewarding service opportunities for me have been those that not only fulfilled me personally and professionally but also made a lasting impact on the community.

The Risk of Overcommitment

Have you ever heard the phrase "Too much of a good thing is bad"? Well, this can be true for service and academic citizenship. Service is great and can be fun, but not when you overdo it and have little time for anything else in your life. I have developed a strategy that helps me remain relevant with my service yet prevents me from overcommitment. I call this strategy conscientious offloading.

Conscientious Offloading

Conscientious offloading is a principle that says before you accept a new opportunity, adequately review your current commitments, and decide which one you are consciously and conscientiously willing to offload (i.e., let go) to create room for the new opportunity.

The word *conscientious* means "wishing to do what is right, especially to do one's work or duty well and thoroughly" (Lexico, n.d.). When you utilize this principle, you are intentionally evaluating your life to be sure you are doing everything well and thoroughly. If you do not exercise conscientious offloading, your plate soon fills up and starts to run over—and not in a good way. Failing to do this is a great recipe for premature burnout in academia, especially when you are first starting your career. Protect your time and mental space, and you will find more meaning and purpose in your work versus doing things because you must.

Last year, I was elected to serve on the board of a professional organization and had taken on other service obligations at the college level. I knew that I could not take on the additional responsibilities of board membership and leadership of another committee at work. I took inventory and asked myself which opportunities would be easier to hand over to someone else and which would provide the best opportunities for both personal and professional growth and needed to be maintained. I decided I would let go of one program at work that I was spearheading. I was passionate about it and was one of the people who built the program from the ground up. But I felt confident that I could ask someone else to lead that program who was equally passionate about its continued success.

I also had to let go of a service commitment with another professional organization. I had served about two years in that capacity, and my letting go gave someone else who was just coming up in their professional career the opportunity to take over. These were important decisions that I needed to make. I could have chosen to maintain the other service obligations, but guess what? I would have been stretching myself too thin, and I would not have been able to devote the necessary attention and effort to all the service opportunities.

The alternative would have been to give all these organizations and committees my very best but fail to take care of my personal needs and well-being, which is equally detrimental. I had to practice conscientious offloading, and I'm glad I did. I must admit that I did not do this well early in my career. As a result, I had time for everyone and everything but not for me. I quickly realized that this was not sustainable and changed course. I had to accept and agree with Tasheka Cox (2019) that self-care is not selfish.

Calculating Distribution of Effort

Another strategy to prevent overcommitment to service opportunities is to calculate the number of hours you spend on service opportunities and compare it with your distribution of effort (DOE) for your specific academic appointment. We discussed this in detail in Chapter 1. Ask yourself a very important question: How much effort do I need to allocate to service based on my academic appointment? This is what should determine how much time you are spending on service opportunities. It has nothing to do with the quality or quantity of the service you are providing—it is strictly about how much *contact time* you spend engaging in your service obligations. I provided an example of an academic appointment that is 60% research, 30% teaching, and 10% service and academic citizenship. The expectation is for you to spend approximately 10% of your time and effort on service opportunities, which amounts to about four hours out of your 40-hour workweek, or about 16 to 20 hours every month.

You can use DOE to estimate whether you are overcommitting by examining how many contact hours in a week or a month you are spending on service opportunities. For example, the following table shows that if my DOE was what was provided in the example, I would be exceeding the expectation for how much time I should be spending on service opportunities. If my DOE for service was 20%, this would definitely be appropriate. Any additional service opportunities would realistically push you into the realm of overcommitment.

Table 4.1 is a sample calculation of service commitment contact hours. This can be useful when determining a realistic service commitment.

TABLE 4.1   SERVICE COMMITMENT CONTACT HOURS

Service Opportunity	Approximate Number of Hours per Month
College Service	
Faculty Organization	2
Undergraduate Faculty Committee	1
Undergraduate Education Committee	1
Graduate Faculty Committee	1
Faculty Life Committee and Subcommittees	1
Undergraduate Peer-Mentoring Program	2
Scholarly Affairs Committee	1
Formal and Informal Mentoring of Faculty	2
Formal and Informal Mentoring of Students	5
University Service	
Core Curriculum Oversight Committee	1.5
Committee on University Committees	1.5
Behavioral Health Conference Planning Committee	1

continues

TABLE 4.1 SERVICE COMMITMENT CONTACT HOURS (CONT.)

Service Opportunity	Approximate Number of Hours per Month
Professional Service	
Sigma Local Chapter	1
Southern Nursing Research Society	3
American Psychiatric Nurses Association	2
American Society of Addictions Nursing	1
International Organization of African Nurses	2
Manuscript Reviews for Various Journals	2
Community Service	
Local Church Volunteering	4
Total	35

Using the template provided in Appendix C, calculate how many contact hours per month you spend on your various commitments. Take into account your service for the college, university, professional organizations, and community. How many contact hours are you spending each month on these opportunities? This is not based in science; it is just my recommendation based on my own experiences and conversations with other faculty members. Anything more than 35 to 40 hours per month of service contact hours starts to stretch you in ways that prevent you from giving your best to each of the opportunities. Now, everyone is different, and some people can handle more than others. Therefore, you have to decide early in your career what you are capable of handling based on your other commitments, the time you have, the resources available to you, and the usefulness of the opportunities in propagating your career forward. What is that number for you?

Prioritizing the Right Type of Service for You

Up to this point, I have given you good reasons why you should not engage in too much service. Now I would like to focus on why you should engage in the *right* types of service opportunities for your career trajectory.

One of the best pieces of advice I received from my mentor when I first started my academic position was to be selective in the types of service opportunities I took on. It was not that I should completely stay away from it unless it was mandatory; her advice was that I should be strategic in what I chose to be a part of. She could not have been more right. What she advised was that I needed to choose service opportunities that complemented my research and scholarship endeavors as well as my teaching obligations. When you do this, you enrich your experiences through the synergistic effects of your complementary endeavors.

The problem, as Heather Pfeifer (2016) notes, is that we have traditionally given people the wrong advice, which is to stay away from service, period. However, this stymies personal and professional progression both in academia and beyond. These misperceptions have stemmed from lack of clarity from institutions regarding the definition of academic citizenship and how it is evaluated. How do we fix this? I believe we do so by highlighting the benefits of service and academic citizenship.

Pfeifer (2016) lists important benefits of academic citizenship, including:

- Broadening of professional skills related to how institutions operate and how they are governed
- Providing opportunities for collaboration and networking
- Advancing your discipline and the quality of the organizations you belong to
- Growing your professional knowledge and expertise, which may help to establish you as an expert in a particular area

- Remaining in touch with the needs of your community and being considered a friend of the community

Final Thoughts

As we close this chapter, I want to emphasize that there are many benefits to academic citizenship and service. You should not completely avoid it. You should, in fact, seek opportunities that are relevant for your professional and personal growth. Be careful, however, not to overcommit; if you are not going to do it well, it is not worth doing. If you overcommit, you will soon get a reputation for not being dependable. Your reputation will precede you, whether in a positive or negative light. Service, if properly done, can be a strategic tool for networking and growing your professional identity. It will help you slowly grow your expertise in many areas, and that will set you up for success in the long run.

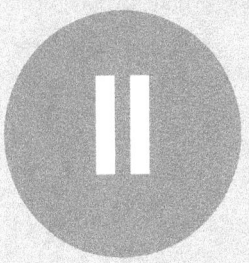

CHOOSING THE BEST ROLE FOR YOU

5   So You've Chosen Tenure Track: Finding the
    Right College for You........................95

6   Becoming a Nurse Researcher and Scientist...115

7   Considerations for Transitioning to a Clinical
    Faculty Role..................................141

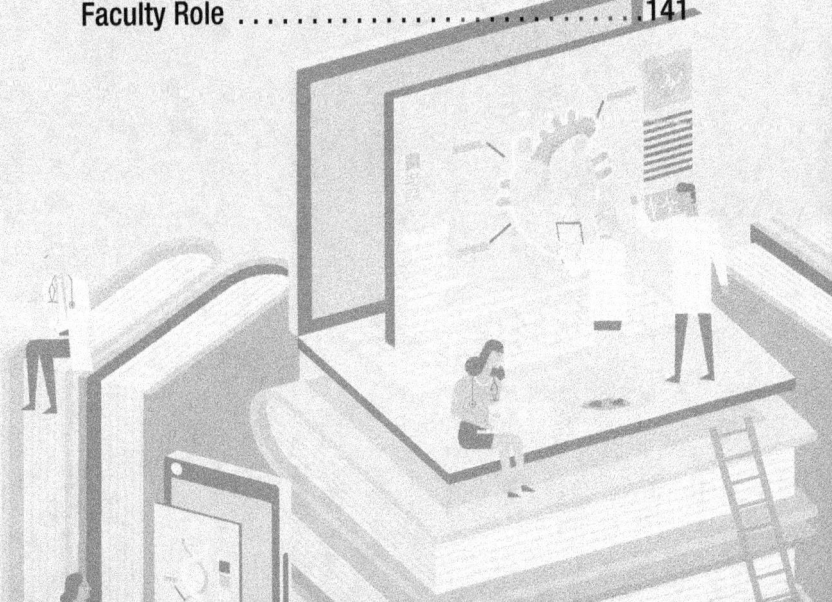

5

SO YOU'VE CHOSEN TENURE TRACK: FINDING THE RIGHT COLLEGE FOR YOU

The first question I usually ask when people tell me they are on tenure track or are thinking about tenure track is why they chose or are considering this path.

You will be surprised at how many people say, "Well, that was the only option I had," or "My mentors told me that is the type of position I should pursue," or even, "It's the only way I will get job security in academia."

These may be logical reasons to choose tenure track, but they should not be the only ones. Why do I say this? Tenure track is often difficult and demanding. Having a bigger "why" will keep you motivated while you paddle your way through the bureaucracies and politics that often plague tenure-track positions.

History of Tenure Track

A little bit of history here. Tenure is an ancient concept that was first developed over a century ago by the American Association of University Professors (AAUP) Committee on Academic Freedom and Academic Tenure (n.d.). They developed a statement that came to be known as the 1915 Declaration of Principles, and it was adopted by the association at the end of its second annual meeting in 1916. In 1925, this statement was revised and shortened by the American Council on Education and then endorsed by AAUP in 1926.

In 1940, however, AAUP and the Association of American Colleges (now the Association of American Colleges and Universities) reevaluated the key policy statements to formulate interpretations of the original statement and to *adapt* it to the needs of that time. The intent of tenure was to promote academic freedom of faculty members and to protect them from unnecessary firing and retribution.

I have emphasized the word adapt because I believe one of the reasons you hear horror stories about tenure track these days is that most universities have failed to do what the faculty and administrators of 1940 did—adapt the expectations and obligations of tenure-track faculty to a consistently changing academic environment. In the late 1930s, Harvard University introduced the concept of emphasizing research for those on tenure track, and universities across the country followed suit over the coming years. Although other models of promoting other institutional priorities have been implemented, nothing has significantly changed related to expectations of tenure-track faculty (Worthen, 2021).

This lack of adaptability has led to frustration, power struggles, insensitivities, and sheer lack of understanding of the personal needs of individuals on tenure track, which often leads to a culture of do or die (Carr, 2014). Some people thrive in these types of conditions, and that is wonderful, but for most of us, this environment is highly unsustainable and leads to high attrition rates among those choosing this type of academic appointment. In fact, the percentages of tenure-track and tenured professors in both public and private universities have been steadily declining since the 1970s (AAUP, 2006).

According to the 1940 Statement of Principles of Academic Freedom and Tenure, tenure is:

> A means to certain ends; specifically: (1) freedom of teaching and research and of extramural activities, and (2) a sufficient degree of economic security to make the profession attractive to men and women of ability. Freedom and economic security, hence, tenure, are indispensable to the success of an institution in fulfilling its obligations to its students and to society. (AAUP, n.d., para. 8)

Because tenure promises freedom and security, many of us are eager to sign up for a probationary period that some describe as servitude because of the conditions usually associated with this path. For example, some universities will terminate your probationary period if you fail to meet the demands of the appointment, which often means leaving the academic unit or even the institution.

This do-or-die pervasive culture is known to cause serious anxieties among individuals on tenure track and, if not handled well, can lead to mental health challenges (Academia, 2013; Carr, 2014; Lashuel, 2020). I have noticed that this culture can further perpetuate unhealthy competition among individuals on tenure track, who may feel that they are competing for the same resources, opportunities, and even recognition. This unhealthy competition, if not properly addressed by the college administrators, may lead to sabotage, which fosters a survival-of-the-fittest attitude among individuals on tenure track.

But it doesn't have to be that way. To counteract this culture, the American Council on Education (n.d.) developed a comprehensive report, "An Agenda for Excellence: Creating Flexibility in Tenure-Track Faculty Careers," which calls on all university presidents and chancellors to act now to improve conditions for tenure-track faculty. Therefore, ensuring that you are accepting a tenure-track position at a university or college that meets your career objectives; has a culture that promotes diversity, equity, and inclusion; and promotes work-life balance is foundational to promoting your health and well-being. This is why where you start matters!

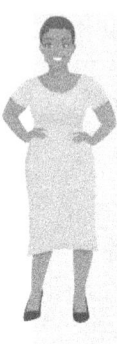

MERCY'S MOMENTS

You might say, "Mercy, all of this sounds horrible! Why should I subject myself to this?" Every university is different. Therefore, do your research. I chose the tenure-track route because of its focus on research and scholarship. I love teaching, and in fact, colleagues and students have told me on several occasions that I am an excellent teacher. From the time I started working as a graduate teaching assistant (GTA) and as an adjunct instructor while in my PhD program, my student evaluations have been overwhelmingly positive.

Several students have commented on how much they appreciate my teaching and the way I relate to them—how I simplify complex concepts and support their personal and professional growth. But what I love more is doing research and adding to the scientific body of knowledge for my discipline and profession. So, I chose tenure track because it allowed me protected time to do research and grow as a scientist—and, of course, the promise of academic freedom and job security. This is why I asked you in the beginning what your real "why" is for being on tenure track.

However, simply knowing your why and having a deep understanding of your career objectives do not shield you from potential negative experiences of being on tenure track. Let's dive into your strategic decision-making process and what factors you should consider when applying for a tenure-track position. Or, if you are already on tenure track and feel like you are running a bit off course, I will discuss some strategies to get you back on track. It's never too late to chart a new course.

Factors to Consider When Choosing a College of Nursing

The first things you should consider when deciding whether to accept a tenure-track position are the policies and procedures governing tenure and promotion both at the college level and the institutional level. These policies and procedures will provide guidelines and metrics on what is considered sufficient progress for each category you will be evaluated on—research and scholarship, teaching, and service and academic citizenship.

As you evaluate prospective institutions, keep the following questions in mind.

What Are the Institutional Research Expectations?

The governing policies and procedures for promotion and tenure are often guided by the research classifications of your institution, such as the Carnegie Classification of Institutions of Higher Education (n.d.). Most universities strive to either obtain or maintain the very high research activity designation; but with this comes pressure on faculty, especially those who are on tenure track, to contribute to the research strategic goals and mission in what sometimes seems like a barter system. You give me research and scholarship productivity; I give you tenure and promotion.

Usually, research and scholarly expectations are highly correlated to the research ranking of the university in question. For example, the expectations for tenure and promotion at a highly ranked research university may be five to seven published manuscripts per year, a large federal grant, and an expectation that a certain percentage of your salary will be covered by sponsored programs. On the other hand, the expectations for tenure and promotion at a research institution not ranked as highly may be two to four publications per year and any type of internal or external grant to support your program of research, among others.

What you need to ask yourself is where you feel you can realistically achieve or even exceed the expectations as set forth by the tenure and promotion policies and procedures. There is no right or wrong answer. This is an individual decision and should be based on what you feel you can commit to while maintaining all other aspects of your life.

MERCY'S MOMENTS

When I was finishing my PhD program, I looked at several universities and their requirements for tenure and promotion. I also tried to talk to people who were either currently on tenure track at those institutions or had received tenure and promotion. It was evident to me that experiences vary widely depending on where you chose to start your career. For me, it was not only about the experience I would have, nor the prestige associated with the university, but also about the support and infrastructure available to help me reach my personal objectives for growth and development. Notice I said my personal objectives. While my work would support the mission and agenda of the university I chose, it was important to me that the position would provide the foundation and infrastructure for me to grow and develop in ways that were personally meaningful.

I like to think of myself as a highly motivated individual who will rise to the challenge of whatever is placed in my way. But I intentionally avoided starting my tenure-track position at a very highly ranked research university because I wanted to have a life outside of my work once I was done with school. This may not sound very ambitious, but that was how I felt. I went to school full time and worked full time while I was working on my PhD. On average, I slept four to six hours a night for the four years I was in my doctoral program. To say that I was exhausted by the time I was done would be an understatement. I was burned out. And on top of that, I had a really bad experience with one of my professors who literally did not believe that I was "PhD material," whatever that meant. I needed to reclaim and bring a bit more sanity into my everyday life. Therefore, starting a position at an institution where I was expected to publish five to seven manuscripts a year and get an R01 National Institutes of Health (NIH) grant before I could apply for promotion and tenure was off the table. I'm not saying there is anything wrong with that; it just wasn't right for me.

I love writing and disseminating my research. I can hit those benchmarks, but I did not want to feel like I always had something hanging over my head. On average, I publish four to seven articles in peer-reviewed scientific journals every year, and I have been blessed to secure multiple large grants totaling over $9 million as principal investigator and over $17 million overall since starting tenure track five years ago. But I reach these benchmarks because I'm passionate about my work, not because I *must* do them to keep my job. Therefore, my first rule of thumb on thriving and not merely surviving on tenure track is that you choose a university that has tenure and promotion expectations you can realistically meet without sacrificing your personal health and mental well-being in the process.

What Supports Are Offered?

The next thing to consider about where to start your tenure-track position is the infrastructure that is available to support your growth and development as an emerging scholar. This may include a dedicated office or department to support research and scholarship needs of faculty, a full-time dean of research, graduate student support, and availability of startup research funds or ongoing internal seed funding to support pilot projects as you begin to develop your program of research. This is very important because most people who are starting tenure-track positions are fresh out of their doctoral program and may have had limited research experience in their program.

Doctoral programs differ in their capability to prepare their graduates to transition into research-intensive positions soon after graduation. Being honest about your research abilities, needs, and opportunities is very important in determining what infrastructure and support you will need to hit the ground running as you begin your tenure-track position. Before you start, you must ask the right questions to ensure these supports are available to you; otherwise, you will be setting yourself up for failure, especially if the doctoral program you graduated from does not have high research productivity expectations for its students.

Many research-focused nursing doctoral programs are moving toward providing their students with research experiential opportunities to lessen the potential for failure among those pursuing tenure-track positions after graduation. If you feel you did not have strong research preparation in your doctoral program but still want to pursue a tenure-track position, there are several things you can do to bridge the knowledge–experience gap and be successful in establishing yourself as an independent researcher.

Additional supports might include the presence of a center for research in your chosen trajectory, a center for clinical and translation science, research institutes that provide collaborative platforms for multidisciplinary teams across campus, and a very engaged institutional office of research and development. Remember that your needs are unique, and you need to ensure that the infrastructure to support your personal growth as a scientist is available at the institution you are considering.

In Chapter 3, I talked about doing a SWOT analysis. I recommend that you do one specifically related to your research and scholarship goals and objectives so that you can determine how best to leverage the resources and supports at your institution. Another strategy I recommend if you feel you didn't have a strong research experiential background in your doctoral program is to enroll into research training programs that will help you sharpen your skills in a desired area.

In fact, this is also true when you need to acquire new skills that will be relevant to developing and growing a new aspect of your research trajectory. I will talk more about this in Chapter 6. Seeking additional research training before you begin tenure track or early in your journey may prove helpful in ensuring your long-term success, even beyond the probationary period.

> **SUCCESS NUGGET**
>
> Seeking additional research training before you begin tenure track (such as a postdoctoral fellowship) or early in your journey may prove helpful in ensuring your long-term success, even beyond the probationary period.

What Are Other Faculty Members Working On?

The next point of consideration is to evaluate the types of research that current faculty members are doing at that college or even the university. This is very important when you are starting out because you need to quickly develop your program of research, which will be propagated if other people within the college or university are already doing similar work. Some of my colleagues have turned down great opportunities because no one was doing research that would remotely support their programs of research at the institution that was trying to recruit them. A college may be unable to provide infrastructure required to do a specific type of research—for example, if you need certain equipment that is not already available, and the college is not able to secure it for you. The logistical nightmare of having to go to a lab in a different town or state may not be worth everything else being offered for you to take that position.

What Is the Culture Surrounding Research and Scholarly Productivity?

The college's culture regarding research and scholarly productivity should also be evaluated. If you are considering a teaching-intensive university to begin your tenure-track career, I caution you to manage your expectations related to teaching and service requirements. These institutions have a heavy focus on teaching, but they may also have lower expectations for research and, inadvertently, poor support for individuals on tenure track. I advise you to go into this type of institution with eyes wide open. Because the institution is heavily focused on teaching, other faculty who are not on tenure track may feel that you get preferential treatment when you get course releases for research. Although more institutions are striving to have a greater focus on research and scholarly productivity, institutions that previously focused only on teaching may still exhibit a culture that is not very welcoming to research-focused faculty. Understanding the college and institutional culture will help you make informed decisions about joining the college and will help you manage your expectations related to appreciation of research and scholarly productivity.

Does the Institution Have Adequate Intramural Seed Funding?

The last important consideration in choosing a college is availability of intramural seed funding to support pilot work for new investigators. *Intramural seed funding* is funding that is available to faculty within an organization to support their research and scholarly activities. I'm basing this question not on scientific data but rather personal observations and anecdotal experiences. There are very few doctorally prepared nurses who come into a tenure-track position having already received funding for any type of research. In fact, several doctoral programs that I know of do not even have grant writing as a course in their curriculum. It may just be a concept that is interwoven into other courses. Sometimes it puzzles me how we expect people to suddenly be able to acquire internal grant funding, let alone external grant funding, if we are not giving them these basic tools in our doctoral programs. (I address this in more detail in Chapter 6.)

Furthermore, most external funding agencies want to see that individuals have previously conducted funded work, even if it is a pilot study. The exception is external grant funding opportunities that are specifically designed for new investigators needing seed funding to jumpstart their program of research, such as those from professional organizations and some foundations. With this reality in mind, institutions with robust intramural funding opportunities are preferable to those that do not have this infrastructure in place. This point goes hand in hand with the overall university infrastructure to support new investigators on tenure track.

> **SUCCESS NUGGET**
>
> As you develop as a scientist, you will appreciate that sometimes less can be more. When you have access to seed funding that you can use to conduct smaller pilot and feasibility studies, you will be better prepared to acquire larger grants later in your career because you have established a reputation of developing, conducting, and completing smaller grant projects. It's even more important to aim for dissemination of findings from your smaller grants as this will give funders more confidence in your ability to successfully complete future studies.

Does the Institution Offer Access to an Established Scientist in Your Field Who Could Serve as a Mentor?

Understanding whether your college or institution has senior scientists with similar research interests who could potentially serve as mentors is important. I recommend securing a highly productive and well-established mentor in your research area of interest whenever possible. Most of the time, the expectation is that individuals slowly transition from mentored research to independent research by the time they are going up for tenure and promotion. When you align yourself with a mentor who has an established program of research, you not only receive mentorship benefits but quickly begin to grow your own associated, but independent, program of research.

Additionally, highly productive mentors are often looking for eager, enthusiastic junior faculty to help their research labs run smoothly. This quickly teaches you about team dynamics, leadership of research teams, and management of graduate research assistants (GRA) or other affiliated personnel. Volunteering to take the load off your mentor provides you experiential research opportunities that you otherwise may not have access to. Therefore, access to established scientists in your field should be a major consideration in choosing a college or institution. This person does not necessarily have to be in your college of nursing.

MERCY'S MOMENTS

When I was in my PhD program, I worked as a GRA in the Center for Research and Scholarship. I liked this experience because it provided me with hands-on training for conducting research on human subjects and allowed me to work with various professors in the college of nursing who had diverse programs of research. So, coming into the tenure-track position, I felt very confident in my ability to conduct research and transition to an independent researcher. I soon realized that being a part of a research team is quite different from building and leading a research team. I acknowledged my weaknesses in this area and decided to seek out mentorship specifically related to building and leading multidisciplinary, highly productive teams.

At the time, I had a dual appointment with the local Veterans Affairs Medical Center (VAMC), and my mentor was the Associate Chief of Research and Development at that VAMC. I told her that I felt I was weak in this area, but my goal was to build a robust and sustainable program of research that was maintained by a highly productive, multidisciplinary team of investigators and collaborators. I did not want to be just a stellar solo scientist. I wanted to make sure that my work would have long-term impact and be highly significant. Thankfully, she was kind enough to take me under her wing and teach me everything she knew about building and leading research teams—and I'm still learning.

As you can see, my biggest needs were not related to publication help or hands-on training; I felt like I had that foundation. But to elevate the quality of my work, I needed to seek out a mentor who had a proven record of building and leading research teams and departments. What is your biggest mentoring need? The answer to this question will inform your next steps in looking for appropriate mentorship to grow as a scientist and transition to independent research.

Let's say that your biggest need is related to publication success. Highly productive mentors may have a backlog of manuscripts that they need to send out for publication. You can offer to help with developing those manuscripts and negotiate authorship with them. Sometimes, they have so much data from completed and ongoing studies that you can obtain expedited institutional review board (IRB) approval to conduct secondary data analyses, thereby giving you the opportunity to quickly churn out data-based manuscripts as first author. I will talk more about how to leverage your relationship with your research mentor in Chapter 6. Again, an important consideration for where you elect to start your tenure-track position is whether you have mentoring support within your college or opportunities to seek out mentors outside of your college.

How Does the Dean of Research Support Faculty?

The last strategy is that you need to do your own homework related to the type of dean of research you will be working with. When you interview for tenure-track positions, you often have a separate interview with the college's dean of research. In my opinion, outside of meeting with the dean and faculty, this will give you the most important insights into your potential for success on tenure track. When you are on tenure track, you can be the best teacher on the planet, but if you are not meeting your research and scholarship expectations, you will not be promoted or receive tenure. Therefore, making sure that you have a supportive dean of research will be instrumental to your success.

I was very fortunate when I started my tenure-track position that I had a dean of research who understood my individual needs and connected me to resources and potential collaborators on campus.

To this day, the people she introduced me to are some of my most dependable team members. Therefore, make your dean of research your most valuable resource. Their role is to help you be successful.

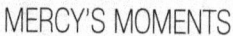

MERCY'S MOMENTS

A lot of people are surprised that I was able to secure large National Institutes of Health (NIH) funding as a principal investigator very early in my career. The secret to this success, I believe, was the infrastructure available at my institution that exposed new investigators to the inner workings of the NIH and fostered personal connections between investigators and program officers. I will talk more about making your program officer your best friend in Chapter 6. But I want to underscore that if I had not been exposed to the NIH in meaningful ways at a very early stage in my career, I would probably still be thinking that I was not ready to submit a proposal to the institute for funding consideration.

At my university, investigators who want to submit a proposal to the NIH work with their dean of research to identify an appropriate parent announcement (PA) of request for application (RFA) from the NIH. After this, they develop a competitive specific aims page for their proposed project. Once the specific aims are reviewed and approved by a select panel in the university's Office of Research and Development (ORED), the investigators then work with their dean of research to contact the appropriate program officer (PO) to schedule an appointment. The investigators send the PO their specific aims page at least two weeks in advance. On the agreed date, the university flies a group of investigators and their deans of research to Washington, DC, to meet in person with the program officers—in a private jet I might add.

During that meeting, the junior faculty member has the opportunity to ask appropriate questions, and the dean for research provides support and ensures that other questions that the investigator may not even have thought about are also brought up to and addressed by the PO. I cannot tell you how valuable this experience was for me. I participated in this program twice, and both my trips were meaningful and yielded significant outcomes for my research trajectory.

During both trips, the PO generously introduced me to other POs in case I decided to take my proposal in a different direction. They even suggested appropriate study sections that I could request to review my proposals. Up to this point, I did not know this was a possibility. The only expectation my university had was that I would submit a full proposal to the NIH within a year of my trips. I share this story to simply underscore the emphasis of this chapter—it matters where you start your career as a tenure-track faculty member because that plays a big role in how successfully you navigate this process.

Falling Behind

You might be saying, "Mercy, this is all great advice, but I did not consider these issues before I started my tenure-track position, and I'm not making the type of progress that I need to be making. It is too late for me?" The answer to your question depends on the circumstances. If you are still early within your probationary period (less than three years), there might be room to get back on course. This is highly dependent on what you have accomplished so far and how far you are from meeting the expectations for tenure and promotion based on your institution's policies and procedures.

Scenario 1: I'm Behind on Publication Requirements

Let's say the publication requirement for promotion and tenure at your institution is an average of three publications as first or second author every year, with a minimum of 12 peer-reviewed publications as first or second author to be considered for tenure and promotion at the end of your mandatory review year. You are in your third year of tenure track and still have three years to go. If you have consistently published two manuscripts a year up to this point, you could catch up with your required publications during the next three years. However, if you were averaging only one published manuscript per year, that would be a harder climb, and you have to evaluate your priorities—whether to not have much of a life for the next three years and hopefully get back on track or look at alternatives.

Alternatives would depend on many factors. For example, if your success as a teacher and mentor to students has added significant value to the university or college, you might be able to discuss with your dean the possibility of seeking promotion without tenure or leaving tenure track and moving to an instructor or clinical assistant professor position. Both of these options are highly dependent on the culture at your university or college and how these types of situations have been handled in the past, which established precedence. Another option would be to consider transferring to another institution with less stringent criteria for tenure and promotion (if tenure is important to you) or a clinical track position that has minimal expectations for research and scholarly productivity.

Scenario 2: I'm Falling Behind in Teaching and Research

The second scenario might be that you are struggling to meet expectations for both teaching and research. In this case, the options might be fewer. It may be in your best interest to be proactive in having conversations with your dean. If there is an opportunity to be retained in a different capacity, and you would like to stay with the college, that should be your first choice. If this is not an option, the fundamental question in seeking opportunities elsewhere would be whether you would like to move to another tenure-track position at a less research-intensive university or you don't want a tenure-track position at all.

Most universities will accept some or all years that you served on tenure track at a different institution, provided you have sufficient evidence of progression toward tenure based on their policies and procedures governing tenure and promotion. Therefore, you should not be afraid of moving to another institution if you feel that will give you a better chance of being promoted and securing tenure. Unfortunately, even if the current institution is not a good fit, many people keep pushing themselves, playing the catch-up game until it's too late to salvage any possibility of tenure and promotion from other institutions. Most of us don't like change, but sometimes change is necessary to make sure you have work-life balance.

Sometimes, you may realize that tenure track is really not for you. And that's OK too. Choosing to go a different path and being happy with yourself are more important than staying in a position where you are miserable. As the saying goes, do not merely exist, live!

Special Considerations for Minority and Foreign-Born Faculty

I love academia. But academia has a long history of othering and discrimination against minoritized groups. For the purpose of this discussion, I am specifically addressing foreign-born faculty members who either moved to the United States to take an academic job, or those who moved to the United States as adults and pursued an academic role. Sometimes the cultural differences can cause a foreign-born faculty member to be perceived as incompetent or inadequate. Additionally, this transition can be difficult because the faculty member must learn about the culture of the country as well as the organization, while at the same time managing their own transition into the academic role. One of my mentors, Dr. Stacciarini, recounts her experience of transitioning into an academic role in an article she published two years after moving to the United States from Brazil. In this article, she recounts the major transition milestones and offers strategies on a successful transition, including making information readily accessible to new foreign-born faculty, avoiding colloquialism when communicating, and being assigned a mentor to help with the transition period (Stacciarini, 2002).

Unfortunately, as minority or foreign-born faculty, you are exposed to additional inequities during the tenure and promotion process that white counterparts don't even have to think about. These inequities are well documented. Because of these inequalities, minority faculty attrition is high, they are less likely to be promoted or to receive tenure, and often receive teaching overloads compared to their white counterparts (Abelson et al., 2018; Fang et al., 2000; Peterson et al., 2004). As long as people in academia continue to ignore these ills and act like everyone is treated fairly, minority and foreign-born faculty will continue to get the short end of the stick, and nothing will change.

I was oblivious to these inequities, so imagine my surprise when two months into starting my tenure-track position, a colleague gave me a book by Kerry Ann Rockquemore and Tracy Laszloffy titled *The Black Academic's Guide to Winning Tenure—Without Losing Your Soul* (2008). I asked her why she gave me this book in particular, and she said, "Because you're gonna need it!" At first, I did not understand, but as I read the book, I realized that I was gaining knowledge and skills that would help me be successful on tenure track. Topics explored in the book include understanding race, power, and the academic institution; the politics of "fit"; and the importance of shifting from habits of survival to strategies of success as a Black faculty member.

As I read through this book, it felt like a double whammy for me because I was considered a minority faculty member and was foreign-born. Understanding the intersectionality of race and power in the academic setting made me aware of potential pitfalls; thus, I armed myself with tools and strategies to maintain my integrity while being successful with tenure track. I highly recommend this book, not just for Black faculty but any faculty member who identifies with minority groups, as it addresses many cross-cutting issues.

I bring this up because if you are a minority or foreign-born faculty member, you may find yourself in a college that does not value diversity, equity, inclusion, and belonging (DEIB). I wish this was not the case, but we have to acknowledge that these issues exist. I recommend that you do your due diligence in understanding your college's and institution's stance on issues pertaining to DEIB.

Important questions to ask include:

- Are there policies and procedures governing such issues?
- Does the college specifically address DEIB priorities within the strategic plan?
- How are these priorities actualized?
- Does the executive council have an administrative role specific to DEIB?
- What are the experiences of minority faculty members in that college?

While institutions can make these issues priorities on paper, the actual experiences of minority groups might be different. My recommendation is that you request to speak with a couple of minority faculty as part of your interview process and have genuine conversations about their experiences within the college or the institution at large.

Chapter 8 will take a closer look at academia through the lens of diversity, equity, inclusion, and belonging.

SUCCESS NUGGET

As a minority faculty, you need to be acutely aware of the ways in which inequities in academia are perpetuated through structural and institutional racism. Familiarizing yourself with these practices will allow you to adequately advocate for yourself and others. It is often said that what you don't know won't hurt you, but that is not true when it comes to DEIB experiences of minority faculty at academic institutions. Knowledge will empower you to be proactive and make informed choices about whether or not to join the institution.

Final Thoughts

Tenure track can be a challenging experience for many faculty members. Being proactive in choosing the right college based on your personal and professional objectives will help you set yourself up for success. In this chapter, we have explored not only the important questions you need to ask as you consider an institution but also how to correct your course if you find yourself falling behind. Tenure track can be a worthwhile experience and an important catalyst to your growth as a scientist. Having the right resources, infrastructure, and support can lead to your exponential growth and quickly establish you as a developing scientist in your field.

6

BECOMING A NURSE RESEARCHER AND SCIENTIST

The process of becoming a nurse researcher and scientist requires strategic, international, and well-thought-out planning. As discussed in Chapter 5, where you start matters, and choosing the right college for your personal and professional career objectives and goals will set you up for success. Chapter 5 focused on what I call *external contributing factors* to your development and success. They provide the necessary infrastructure, environment, and resources necessary for you to begin your journey of transitioning to independent research. While these factors are important, they only complement the *internal contributing factors* to your success—what you do to ensure your own success. That will be the focus of this chapter.

Many things are out of your control when you are on tenure track and begin developing as a scientist. However, a lot of things are still in your control; by focusing your energies on those, you can try to maximize these factors and optimize your outcomes. As Tony Fahkry (2018) says, "Life is not happening to you, but responding to you." Adopting this mindset is crucial; otherwise, you will feel like a victim of circumstances at every turn in your journey to becoming a nurse scientist.

Life responds to what you do. Consider Newton's Third Law of Motion (The Physics Classroom, n.d., para. 2): "For every action, there is an equal and opposite reaction." You will get out of life what you put in, all things being equal. As I discuss various strategies to employ on your journey to become a nurse scientist, you will soon realize that this process can, and should, be enjoyable and worthwhile.

I will take a methodical approach to discuss several internal contributing factors to your success. First, I would like to ask you a simple question: How would you define your program of research?

Defining Your Program of Research

In their book, *Developing a Program of Research: An Essential Process for a Successful Research Career*, Nancy Edwards and Susan Roelofs (2019) propose two guiding principles in selecting and developing your program of research. First, evaluate the state of the science in your current field and the potential for return on investment. In other words, is your research significant, and does it have the potential to generate new knowledge to be added to the body of scientific knowledge in the field? Does it have the potential for sustained impact? These are the "so what" questions. The answers to these questions will assist you in carving out your niche and guide you as you begin the process of becoming an expert in your area of interest.

The second principle focuses on the issue of practicality and addresses the following question: What is the practicality of implementing your program of research based on available infrastructure and human capital? And might I add, what is the congruence with priorities of major funding agencies? While this may not be a major consideration when you are first starting out, as you grow as a scientist, so do the expectations for securing funding to support your program of research. In Chapter 5, I shared with you a story about a colleague who turned down a really great job offer because the university that was trying to recruit her had neither the research infrastructure nor the human capital to support the program of research she wanted to build. It would have been impractical for her to conduct her research if she had moved to that institution. Moreover, it would have significantly stymied her career progression in the long run. The point is, always consider the practicality of the program of research you are trying to build.

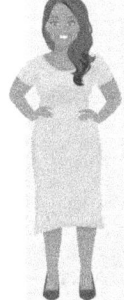

MERCY'S MOMENTS

Truth be told, when I first started my tenure-track job, I didn't even understand the full implications of this type of position. I knew I was passionate, enthusiastic, and eager to do whatever was in my power to grow and develop into a nurse scientist. How that was going to happen, I wasn't very sure. I knew what I needed to do for my annual merit evaluation as well as my tenure and promotion reviews, but I had not yet developed a personal research strategic plan to guide the development and implementation of my program of research.

During one of my initial meetings with my dean of research, she asked me what I thought was a simple question: "How would you describe your program of research?" Of course, I blubbered my way through what I thought was an intelligent answer to her question. Imagine my surprise when she said, "Mercy, you just described a few research studies you are planning to do. That is not your program of research." I was confused! She proceeded to educate me on what she meant by a program of research. That is when it dawned on me. I had ideas of studies I wanted to conduct, but in my mind, they were all independent projects, whose processes of implementation, translation, and dissemination had to be mutually exclusive.

At that time, I hadn't broadened my thinking enough to know how my passions, expertise, state of the science in my field, and funding priorities merged to inform a research strategic plan that would serve as a compass for prioritizing effort, seeking additional resources, training, and expanding collaborations with an ultimate goal—improving patient and population outcomes in my desired area of research. I then realized that more goes into developing a program of research than simply conducting one study after another. So, I pose this question also to you: What is your program of research? Until you can adequately define what it means for you, you cannot create a research strategic plan that includes specific and measurable goals supported by corresponding objectives and related tasks to actualize your identified goals.

Understanding your program of research will further help you remain focused, which allows you to begin establishing yourself as an expert in a particular field. Speaking of expertise—in that same conversation, my dean of research asked me another question: "What do you want to be known for five to 10 years from now? That was simple! I want to be an addictions scientist who helps people recover from substance use disorders and reincorporate into society as productive citizens. "There are a lot of ways to do that," she said, "so what will be your niche?" I hadn't clearly thought this through. Up to this point, I believed that expertise simply comes with time, and that is true.

To become a nurse scientist within a defined program of research that will be nationally and internationally recognized, you must intentionally carve your own space within the broader context of your research area of interest. You will not accidentally become an expert in your field. So, what's your plan to get there? Below we address important considerations for your growth and development as a nurse scientist.

SUCCESS NUGGET

Understanding your program of research will further help you remain focused, which allows you to begin establishing yourself as an expert in a particular field. Additionally, defining your program of research early will help you create a niche that will distinguish you from other scientists within your chosen field of research.

Developing a Strategic Plan

Now that you have defined your program of research and identified your niche, your next step is developing a strategic plan on how to actualize the program of research. Below are important questions to ask yourself in this process, as suggested by Edwards and Roelofs (2019):

- What research design or designs do you plan to use, and are they primarily qualitative, quantitative, or mixed methods?
- What populations do you plan to study?
- What health, societal, or economic issues are of primary interest to you?
- Will your studies be undertaken locally or nationally? Will they span jurisdictions? Will they have a global orientation?
- How will partners such as policymakers, managers, and decision-makers be involved?
- What disciplines do you intend to collaborate with and why?

Take some time to jot down the answers to the questions above. Where you are not sure, can you do some research on what other scientists in your field are doing? Take some time to give two or three rationales about why you have answered a particular question a certain way. Forcing yourself to think through your answers helps you identify your own blind spots on areas that need clarification as well as improvement. If you cannot convince yourself of your intended trajectory, it will be much harder to convince someone else that what you are trying to pursue is worthwhile.

Creating a Research and Scholarship Plan

Part of developing your research strategic plan requires that you create a research and scholarship plan, which serves as the road map to actualize your program of research. It should have pillars that are congruent with the categories of your annual merit evaluation and your promotion and tenure requirements, if applicable. Examples of pillars for your trajectory include publications, grant funding, presentations at research conferences or other dissemination platforms, and other professional activities that contribute to your scientific profile, such as reviewing abstracts for research conferences.

All of these are important; however, there are other pillars that early science investigators often do not consider as they are creating their research and scholarship trajectory. These include involvement and engagement with community stakeholders, the scientific community, and students. Your research strategic plan should have at least three pillars. For example, my personal research strategic plan has five pillars: publications, presentations, grant funding, professional service that complements my research, and community engagement. Below are examples of what I track under each pillar:

Publications

- Number of publications each year
- Target journals to publish in and their corresponding impact factors
- Publication impact metrics, such as number of citations per publication, h-index, and i10-index
- Researchers outside the United States citing my work (for global impact)

Presentations

- Total presentations per year (both peer-reviewed and invited)
- Level of presentations (I like to have a mixture of international, national, regional, and local presentations each year.)

- Invited presentations based on my expertise
- Research seminars developed each year on a specific topic

Grant Funding

- Types of research being funded (e.g., research grants, program grants, or service grants)
- Grant funding sources and goals for diversifying grant funding sources (e.g., NIH, HRSA, SAMHSA, foundation grants)
- Grant projects that are progressing according to timeline (including progress reports and final reports submitted on time)
- Grants that are being completed and results disseminated

I do the same for the other two pillars and make sure that I am meeting my own benchmarks. My personal benchmarks can be similar or different from expectations of my college. They are whatever I think really affords me the opportunity to grow at the rate that matches my abilities and the resources available to me.

At the beginning of every year, I take time to create a plan for that year. Doing so allows me to anticipate deadlines, develop a plan for gathering resources and collaborators to meet my objectives, and gauge what other responsibilities I may need to let go of based on anticipated new activity in the year. Remember conscientious offloading from Chapter 4? Yes, I'm constantly doing that to ensure that I'm not being overcommitted due to lack of planning. So, what are the pillars of your own research strategic plan, and how do you measure success?

FINDING THE RIGHT RESEARCH MENTOR

Research mentors are foundational components of building your program of research. The right mentor will be instrumental in teaching you aspects of being a scientist that are outside the experiential components of conducting research. However, a mentor cannot force you to grow beyond your own desired limits. This is why it is important to set your own personal research goals to ensure that your mentor has metrics to evaluate the success of the mentoring relationship as well. Another important reason to have your own targets and discuss them with your mentor is that sometimes when you are working with highly productive mentors, it is easy to overcommit on research productivity because your mentor is highly successful. Remember you are still developing as a scientist; you may currently not have the capacity to write 10 grants and publish 15 papers each year.

I cannot overemphasize the value of having the *right* mentor for your current season of development. Being honest about your needs will ensure your success in securing the right mentors. Additionally, sometimes it's better to approach a mentor who may not necessarily be at the top of the "food chain" in your field of research, but one who has sufficient expertise and time to mentor you. While it might be a great opportunity to be mentored by the top expert in your field, sometimes this person is so busy—by virtue of being the leading researcher everyone goes to and the added responsibilities that come with prestige and fame—that they may not have the time to give you the individualized attention that you need to build the program of research you envision.

SUCCESS NUGGET

In Chapter 3, we discussed the secrets of networking, and one of the concepts we discussed is adding value to others. Believe it or not, you can add value to your mentor's work in such a way that the relationship is mutually beneficial. This can be as simple as helping with manuscript development, suggesting new ideas and processes (if the mentor is open to suggestions), and being respectful of the networks your mentor allows you to access. This last point is quite important and is often overlooked. It is important to represent mentors well when they provide you the opportunity to connect with someone in their network. You should always strive to represent your mentor in a good light. As I begin to mentor more doctoral students and junior faculty, this principle is becoming even more meaningful to me.

Building Your Research Team

When building a program of research, you quickly learn that leading a research team is very different from being part of a research team. Your long-term success is dependent on your leadership and management capabilities, and this is where your mentor becomes even more instrumental. I shared with you a story in Chapter 5 about how I specifically asked one of my mentors to teach me the ins and outs of managing and leading research teams. This looks easy on the outside, but moving from a one-person show as a mentored scientist to providing a vision and goals around which other investigators, staff, and students can rally requires growth and deliberate effort. Before you start inviting people to your table, make sure that you equip yourself with knowledge and skills to provide strategic leadership so that everyone feels valued and their expertise and contributions are respected.

Many people, including me, talk about building your team as if it should just organically happen. We often tell early-career investigators to build their team but never really show them how to do it. However, there is a *process* to building effective teams. I touched on this a little bit in Chapter 3. Identifying your strengths, weaknesses, opportunities, and threats provides great insights into which areas of your life need fortification. When you determine the areas where you lack expertise, you will know whom you need to have on your team to actualize your vision.

Networking to build collaboration is one important aspect of this process. Sometimes as you build teams, you will have people who have previously worked together on other projects. Although these people may have known each other outside of working with you, when they join your team, they are now specifically working together because of you. You are now the common denominator and have the responsibility to promote common vision. There are certain strategies you can implement to promote common vision and mutual respect. We delve into some of them in the paragraphs that follow.

Assign Specific Roles Based on Expertise

Assign specific roles to your team members based on their expertise. For example, part of my program of research involves training behavioral-health paraprofessionals in our state. A good friend of mine is a curriculum guru, and everyone on our team knows that she is the go-to person for curriculum development and implementation. On the other hand, I have another great colleague and friend who understands program evaluation inside out. Our team knows that if you have questions related to program evaluation, he's the man. However, as the program director, I need to understand team members' strengths and allow them to make significant contributions. They are part of our team because of what they can contribute, not just so we can say our team has people with expertise.

Provide Clear Goals and Objectives

Another strategy is to provide clear goals and objectives that are specific, measurable, and time-based. I find this strategy to be particularly important as you begin to work together as a team to implement certain aspects of your program of research. You have to let people know what you need them to accomplish by a specific date. It goes without saying that you need to give your team members ample time for them to deliver what you are asking for. If you assign tasks at the last minute and expect your staff or collaborators to pretty much abandon their lives to meet *your* goal, their morale goes down, and their respect for you as a leader quickly diminishes. Therefore, as the visionary of the team, you must think ahead and anticipate needs. Understanding what team members will need and the time it will realistically require for them to accomplish a particular task helps them feel valued and builds self-confidence because you are setting them up for success.

Expect the Process to Take Time

The process of building a team takes time—therefore, start as early as possible. Also, remember that your team will go through growing pains; don't be discouraged along the way. In the 1960s, psychologist Bruce Tuckman developed a model that identified the four stages of team building: forming, storming, norming, and performing (Tuckman & Jensen, 1977). As you are building your team, be cognizant of which stage your team is in during the process. This understanding will guide what strategies you utilize to maintain momentum, improve team dynamics, and resolve challenges.

As your teams continue to go through the different phases, several strategies might prove useful in helping you quickly get to the performing stage. These strategies have been beneficial to me:

- Assign roles and responsibilities to everyone on your team. When you get rid of ambiguity in roles and responsibilities, you lessen the potential for team members stepping on each other's toes, thereby avoiding unnecessary conflicts.

- Listen to suggestions, and don't be quick to turn down advice. If your team members feel valued and that their contributions matter, they buy into your vision and will support you. If they feel like it is always about you and what you want, they will stop contributing—not just ideas, but potentially even resources and access to their networks.

- Help your team resolve conflicts whenever possible to restore harmony. Your team members may not always see eye to eye. Remember, you are the common denominator. A house divided against itself will not stand.

- Learn to say thank you. This sounds simple, but it is profound. You will be surprised at how many times people leave teams because they feel unappreciated. When you thank them for doing what perhaps in your mind is just part of their job, they understand that you see the effort they put into the task and that their contributions are important to the successful functioning of the team.

- Do not micromanage people, especially after the team has reached the performing phase. The goal is to build a team that is autonomous and does not need your input for everyday operation. The truth is, as you grow as a scientist, allowing your team members to function autonomously with only periodic check-ins gives you more time to deal with other issues that only you have the authority to handle.

- Schedule regular team meetings to check for progress, resolve issues, and set goals for upcoming reporting periods. Things tend to fall through the cracks when there is no schedule for reporting outcomes. You don't want to find out that something wasn't done a week before your progress report is due to your funding agency. Additionally, having regularly scheduled check-ins promotes accountability and much-needed structure for the team.

- Change your mindset from competition to collaboration. I admit that scientists are competitive by nature, some more so than others. Fight the temptation to compete with your team members. Maintaining a competitive attitude is the quickest way to kill your team.

You Don't Have to "Publish or Perish"

You may have heard the phrase "publish or perish," but I like Tara Gray's (2020) approach of "publish and flourish" better. Academic publishing can be tedious; however, if you learn a few tricks to becoming a prolific writer and scholar, you might just end up loving it. This is what happened to me.

In her book *Publish and Flourish: Become a Prolific Scholar* (2020), Gray gives four recommendations for increasing your writing productivity:

- Writing daily for about 15–30 minutes
- Recording the minutes spent on writing and sharing with your accountability partner
- Writing informally from the first day of the project
- Outlining your manuscript based on an exemplar

Writing daily improves the discipline of writing, makes the task seem doable, and increases productivity over time. Sharing your writing log with an accountability partner improves your own accountability to the process of writing, helps you stay on task, and provides you with a sense of accomplishment for completing a task, which improves self-efficacy in the long run. Writing informally allows you the flexibility to tap into your "writing juices" when they are flowing.

You don't always feel inspired about writing, so when you do, simply type out ideas as they come to you. If you don't initially worry about sources to substantiate what you are saying, you might accomplish more writing in a short amount of time. You can always edit later. Finally, utilizing an outline helps you stay focused and organized in your writing, preventing you from going off on a tangent and wasting time on content that may not make it into your final product.

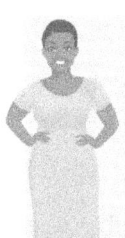

MERCY'S MOMENTS

I loved writing until I enrolled in the PhD program. I was overburdened with paper after paper, and although I was passionate about what I was writing, the pressures of scientific writing took the fun out of it. I knew my tenure-track career would involve a lot of writing. I didn't want to just endure the process; I wanted to enjoy it. After all, I would be doing this for the rest of my life.

I share this story because so many people have told me they do not enjoy writing at all. They would much rather give a presentation about their work and call it a day. And that's fine. In speaking with people about why they hate writing, I have discovered that they may hate the process of writing, but that's only because they do not have the necessary tools to help them boost their productivity, thus making writing a mundane chore.

Another reason people hate writing is that sometimes, early-career scientists focus only on data-based manuscripts to count toward their tenure, to the neglect of other types of publications that can be more fun and contribute to their overall scholarship in meaningful ways. I delve into that later but first, let's look at some strategies that might help you become a prolific writer.

You might say that the recommendation to write every day is a difficult one. It's the one I, too, struggle with the most. I know it works for a lot of people, and much research supports this recommendation. I personally do better when I write in blocks of time. If you are that kind of person, the secret to productivity is to either schedule specific blocks of time on your calendar or to write when you feel most inspired. For me, this block is about three to five hours, depending on what I am working on.

I discovered that I spend a lot of time thinking about what I want to write, creating the outline, and researching content before I actually sit down to write. My writing style feels more like organized chaos—sticky notes everywhere, random notes on grocery store receipts, etc. My husband complains about this because he finds my scribbling all over his paperwork, and he can't figure out what it means. Now he's learned not to throw anything away. By the time I sit down to write, it feels more like a mental dump. This is just how my brain works, and the point is, you have to figure out how you are most productive.

Other strategies that can help make writing for publication more manageable include:

Determine the Time of Day That You Are at Your Best

Another recommendation to increase your productivity is knowing when you are most alert and attentive. This can be early morning for some people, midday for others, or even late at night for night owls. Scheduling your writing time when you are not attentive will just increase your frustration.

Write Other Things

Also, writing about topics that are not as research-focused helps you improve your productivity. You can write about a teaching innovation you implemented, a community project you completed with your students, a commentary or editorial about a prevailing topic in your area of research, and so many more things. In fact, in a special report titled "Scholarship Reconsidered: Priorities of the Professoriate," Ernest Boyer (1990) provides several examples that can serve as a launchpad for academic publications.

Broadening your concept of what you can publish as an early-career scientist is important because other scholarly publications equally contribute to your professional image and profile. If you can free your mind to think creatively about how and what you write, your passion for writing will slowly grow, and you might end up liking the process.

Another reason to explore other forms of scholarly writing is that they are more likely to get published than data-based research manuscripts, which are subjected to a more rigorous review compared to a commentary on a "hot topic." Glanville and Houde (2004) further discuss the benefits of incorporating the scholarship of teaching into your overall research trajectory. They provide examples of activities that you might think relate only to teaching but can be easily converted into publications. These may include topics such as a process you developed to mentor faculty new to the college, an evaluation method you used to assess learner outcomes in your course, and textbooks or book chapters you authored or coauthored. When you are just starting out, every win counts, and the more wins you have, the more confident you become. This ultimately increases your self-efficacy for writing as well as improves the overall quality of your writing.

Form a Writing Team

Utilizing writing teams can further improve your productivity. Writing in groups improves accountability and forces you to adhere to group-established deadlines to submit the scholarly publication for peer review. Furthermore, writing in groups makes the writing process less daunting and may decrease the time it takes to write the manuscript because different people are writing various sections. Moreover, writing in teams gives you the opportunity to learn from others and how they write; allows you to receive peer review before the manuscript is sent out; and enriches the quality of the work because of the diversity of thought, ideas, and experiences that are represented within the writing team. The secret to writing in teams is holding each other accountable; otherwise, there is potential for misunderstanding and frustration when goals and timelines are not clearly communicated or adhered to.

Have Projects at Different Publication Stages

Next, ensure that you have manuscripts in different phases of publication so that you don't have a lapse in your writing—some in the conceptualization stage, some with a few sections written, and others that are almost done and soon will be ready to send out for peer review. This strategy makes writing easier because as you submit one, you have others that with a little extra work will be ready to submit. This strategy prevents you from feeling like you have to start all over again every time you pick up a new manuscript.

Submit Your Work to Journals That Are a Good Fit

The last strategy to increasing your productivity is to submit your work to the right journal. Taking the time to ensure that your manuscript fits within the scope of the target journal is important. Another component of this strategy is to ensure that the target journal doesn't already have a lot of publications related to your topic. A few of my manuscripts were rejected in the past because I submitted them to a journal that had extensively published in that area.

Another tool you can use is a letter to the editor to inquire if they think your work would be of interest to their readership. When you send this letter of inquiry, make sure you include an abstract to provide a comprehensive picture of the work in question.

Use available resources such as Jane (Journal/Author Name Estimator, 2021) to narrow down the journals that would be appropriate for your work. Jane can also help you find potential collaborators by providing authors who have published similar work.

Finally, use your cover letter wisely when you submit your manuscript for publication consideration. Let the editor know how novel your work is, how your findings add to the scientific body of literature, and how the journal readership will benefit from reading your work. Give the editor a good reason why they should consider publishing your work.

Seeking Additional Opportunities for Training

We come out of our doctoral programs with varied research experiences. Becoming a nurse scientist requires you to have many tools in your toolbox. A thorough assessment of your desired additional training will set you up for success. Many early-career scientists have a misconception that participating in additional training will make them appear to be unprepared to operate in their current academic role. To the contrary. As a scientist, you will always be learning new methods, technologies, concepts, etc. Therefore, having a training plan is a major aspect of your development as a scientist and is essential for the growth of your program of research.

SUCCESS NUGGET

As a scientist, you will always be learning new methods, technologies, concepts, etc. Do not shy away from enriching your experiences by participating in various research training programs or even just seminars on emerging topics to keep yourself abreast with the latest evidence in your field.

MERCY'S MOMENTS

When I first moved to Alabama, I was new to the area and not familiar with the region's health disparities or research pertaining to rural communities. However, these two focus areas are an integral part of the university's research program and portfolio. Although my program of research was centered on substance use disorders, I knew that for my work to have the type of impact I wanted, it had to be nested within the context of rural health and health disparities. For that reason, I enrolled in a yearlong fellowship and training program that prepares scientists to conduct rural health and health disparities research. I have never regretted that decision, and I believe it is one of the reasons why I have managed to develop and implement significant programs within our rural communities with far-reaching impact.

I have since participated in three other training programs that I believe were vital to my growth as a scientist: a clinical and translational science training program, a grant-writing training program, and a leadership training program. I also plan to participate in three additional training programs over the next three years that will help me reach the next level of my career as a scientist. Being strategic and intentional in developing a training plan and participating in these types of programs will set you apart from your peers and significantly improve the quality of your work. So, I ask: Do you have a training plan? If not, complete Table 6.1 to create a five-year training plan. Lastly, share your training plan with an accountability partner or mentor to make sure you stay on track with your training.

TABLE 6.1   FIVE-YEAR TRAINING PLAN

	Year 1	Year 2	Year 3	Year 4	Year 5
Focus of Training					
Institution Offering Program					
Applicant Qualifications					
Application Deadline					
Cost of Program					
Benefits of Program					
Resources Needed to Participate					

Strategies to Maximize Grant Funding

In Chapter 5, I discussed the availability of research startup funds and intramural seed funding as a consideration for choosing where you start your career as a nurse scientist, particularly if you are on tenure track. I also mentioned that as an early-career scientist, you may have limited experience writing grants, so you may not be able to secure external funding within the first year of starting your position. That is where research startup funds and internal seed funding play a role in helping you complete smaller studies that will provide the preliminary data you need to apply for larger grants.

However, it may feel like there is an expectation to start working on and securing grants as soon as possible. Securing funding to support your program of research is important, but first you must know how to write a grant proposal. *Grantsmanship*, which Jacob Kraicer (1997, para. 2) defines as "the art of acquiring peer-reviewed research funding," is a significant obstacle for many early-career investigators—whether it's internal seed funding or money from outside sources. Even proficient writers with excellent ideas may struggle with grantsmanship. It also doesn't help when you hear statistics such as average external funding success rates being as low as 10%. Thus, if not addressed, the lack of this particular skill may limit growth as a scientist.

Grantsmanship

When I first started my tenure-track position, I was eager to secure funding for my developing program of research. So, I wrote my first grant. The process at my college was that my dean had to provide a letter of support (LOS) for grant applications. When I sent my grant proposal to the dean as part of my request for the LOS, my dean informed me that it was not ready to be sent to a funding agency. I was crushed. I put my heart and soul into that application, and it felt like rejection. But I understood where she was coming from. If the proposal had no chance to even be reviewed because it was so poorly written, what was the point in submitting it? It wasn't that my proposed research was not novel or significant; it was how the ideas were presented that left my proposal wanting. She recommended that I make a series of appointments with my dean of research, a successful grant writer, to learn grantsmanship from her.

As humbling as this experience was, it was exactly what I needed. It was more important for me to continue perfecting my grantsmanship than to just say I submitted a grant. Unfortunately, early-career investigators sometimes get caught up in the cycle of submitting grants just so they can say they applied, even if the proposal was far from being ready for funding consideration. This often emanates from the constant pressure of performance for those who are on tenure track. The need to be seen doing something not only wastes your valuable time, effort, and resources on something that may not yield the desired effect, but it also diverts your attention from efforts that may provide a better return on investment, such as writing a manuscript.

So, what is grantsmanship, and why does it matter? Kraicer (1997, para. 3) calls the grant application process a competition. I agree that it is truly a competition among scientists to determine who can best convince the funder to support their work. The question still remains—why should your proposal be the one chosen?

Kraicer (1997) also posits: "The art of 'grantsmanship' will not turn mediocre science into a fundable grant proposal. But poor 'grantsmanship' will, and often does, turn very good science into an unfundable grant proposal. Good writing will not save bad ideas, but bad writing can kill good ones" (para. 4).

I couldn't agree more. There are many resources out there on grant writing that might prove useful, but the following strategies may also improve grantsmanship:

- Make sure that your proposed ideas are in line with the funding agency priorities.
- Read all the instructions from the funding agency thoroughly, and ensure that you follow them exactly when preparing your application.

- Develop a specific aims page, and request a meeting with the appropriate funding agency representative to discuss your ideas if that is allowed.
- Provide the significance of your project early in the proposal, and make sure you address the magnitude of the problem you aim to solve.
- Discuss how your proposal is innovative and different from what's already been done.
- Develop a detailed and comprehensive approach section that explains all procedures of how your study will be conducted from start to finish. This may include the study design, recruitment, screening and consenting procedures, randomization procedures (if applicable), data collection and management, statistical analysis plan, personnel responsible for each aspect of the project and required training, and specific and realistic timeline.
- Always have a section for anticipated challenges and how you will resolve them if they arise.
- Utilize the peer-review process prior to submission to the funding agency. Sometimes when you write grants, you start seeing what you want to see. Having someone else with fresh eyes provide feedback will help you polish your proposal and clarify any ambiguities.
- Take a formal grant-writing course (even if you took one in your doctoral program).

Plan How Best to Use Your Research Startup Funds

Research startup funds are an important tool to jumpstart your research trajectory. I suggest that you begin by being strategic with how you use these funds. It is quite temping to use those funds for going to conferences or even a study you have been wanting to do for a while. Before you start spending, go back to how you defined your program of research; you may find that some pilot studies are better to pursue first than others. The question should be based on which ideas will give you the best pilot data to support the next study in the progression of your program of research.

For example, a couple of years ago, I had three ideas related to substance use disorders. On the NIH website, I started looking at the funding priorities for institutes and centers that could potentially fund my research. I noticed that a growing number of RFAs were focusing on medications for opioid use disorders (MOUD). Although I had two other great ideas, I decided to focus my efforts on the pilot study that examined a behavioral intervention to increase adherence to MOUD. Within two years of focusing my efforts on this area within my broad program of research on substance use disorders, I secured a $2.7 million R61/R33 grant from the National Center on Complementary and Integrative Health (NCCIH). Take your time to really think about the best bang for your buck, and don't be in a hurry just to get started.

Establish Yourself as a Member of Your Scientific Community

One of the things that early-career investigators forget to do is to begin establishing themselves as a member of their scientific community. What do I mean by this? I want you to think of the scientific community as a multidisciplinary network of scientists in your field of research. In Chapter 4, I suggested that you need to belong to one professional organization that is specific to your research area of interest but that is not specific to nursing. Beginning to grow your networks outside of nursing will expose you to other opportunities, networks, and resources that you may not otherwise access.

Some of the ways you can do this are to review manuscripts for interprofessional journals, review grants for various funding agencies, attend the professional organization's annual meetings, and volunteer for committees and task forces that are congruent with your research objectives. One opportunity that I recommend for early-career investigators is the Early Career Reviewer Program at the National Institutes of Health. Participating in that program is one of the best decisions I made as an early-career scientist. I believe you will derive the same benefits, including access to other scientists and secrets of the NIH peer-review process. Don't be afraid to get out of your comfort zone.

Evaluating Your Research and Scholarly Productivity

Up to this point, we have talked about ways to develop and sustain your program of research as an emerging scientist. Below is a comprehensive, but certainly not exhaustive, list of ways to evaluate the impact of your research and scholarly productivity. Evaluating the impact of your own work should be a priority to ensure that you are meeting your personal objectives for growth and development. I suggest that you check these metrics every year:

- Number of manuscripts submitted, accepted, and published
- Number of citations from your published works
- Number of grants submitted and funded
- Number of conference abstracts submitted and accepted
- Number of conference abstracts reviewed for other research conferences
- Number of manuscripts reviewed for other scientific journals
- Number of grants reviewed for other funding agencies

- Number of invited presentations
- Number of invitations to serve on boards or committees because of your expertise
- Number and type (local, state, national, international) of media appearances specific to your program of research

Creating a Personal Performance Improvement Plan

In the world of research, things don't always go as planned. And when they don't, you may have to create a personal performance improvement plan (PIP). There are formal ways of creating and developing a PIP when performance is very poor and your employer is considering a formal and legal agreement on how you will improve your performance. That is not what I am discussing here; I am talking about being proactive as a developing scientist and realizing where you are falling short on your personal goals and objectives that you set forth as part of your strategic plan for growing your program of research. I have addressed some ways you can evaluate your own research productivity. If this self-evaluation suggests areas where you could do better, develop a PIP to help you get back on track.

The purpose of the PIP is to provide a detailed plan of how you will remediate the areas where you are falling short. This requires that you identify specific resources and strategies you will employ and people who will assist you with achieving your objectives. The PIP should have a specific time frame in which the issues raised will be addressed and a comprehensive timeline related to each activity you will engage in to improve your performance. Being proactive with this approach will ensure that you are not severely falling behind on your plans for developing into an independent researcher with a robust and sustainable program of research.

Final Thoughts

Becoming a nurse scientist requires intentional and deliberate efforts to develop and implement a program of research supported by targeted strategic planning with specific and measurable goals. This road may be filled with ups and downs and growing pains, but if you persevere and continue to develop your skills, increase knowledge of your field, and establish yourself as a member of your scientific community, you will soon reap the benefits of your hard work. You will make many mistakes. That's OK; let those mistakes teach life lessons that you otherwise may not have learned. I would like to leave you with this quote, often attributed to Nelson Mandela: "It always seems impossible until it is done." So, let's get it done!

CONSIDERATIONS FOR TRANSITIONING TO A CLINICAL FACULTY ROLE

—Whitnee C. Brown, DNP, CRNP, FNP-C, PMHNP-BC

Clinical practice is a pivotal component of being valued as a faculty member, nurse, change agent, and advocate. Professional practice is always evolving, requiring one to reflect on the areas of growth that have been gained with each experience. This growth is vital to the development of future nurses. The clinical expertise gained through years of experience is no small feat. And you should be proud of yourself.

Clinical practice informs nursing education in a myriad of ways; skilled nursing professionals offer feedback, discuss organizational policies, and recommend evidence-based practices to the student population. This skill set qualifies the clinical nursing professional as an extremely valuable asset to academia. Students need to learn safe and equitable patient-centered care, research skills, professionalism, and strategies for quality improvements. Students further need to be prepared for critical review of their performance. Actively practicing in the clinical setting provides premium competency from which students can grow and provides unparalleled clinical mentorship to students.

What to Consider in Clinical Faculty Roles

A clinical faculty role offers the rewarding experience of clinical practice merged with student success, scholarship, and service. The role encompasses leadership, teaching, service, philanthropy, professional development, and initiative. If you are passionate about both teaching and research, academia presents a variety of opportunities. As with any new role, transition can be accompanied by eustress, adaptation needs, uncertainties, and excitement—all rolled into one.

When thinking about the transition into academia, ask yourself, "What are my career intentions? Do I plan to stay in academia long term? Do I like teaching? How much time do I have to contribute? Am I OK with converting from an expert to a novice again? Do I mind being available after hours?" If you answered favorably to the majority of these questions, chances are you will enjoy academia.

As discussed in Chapter 1, the role of the clinical faculty (whether clinical-track assistant professor, instructor, or adjunct) has a greater emphasis on clinical practice and expertise as well as teaching. They are expected to be experts in their chosen field of clinical practice. Traditionally, clinical faculty have the responsibility to adequately prepare students for clinical practice roles. Thus, they tend to have higher teaching loads compared to their tenure-track counterparts.

Again, depending on the specific position type (clinical-track assistant professor, instructor, or adjunct), there may or may not be an expectation for scholarship and conducting research. The courses that clinical faculty teach are dependent on their clinical area of expertise. Thus, clinical faculty with community health nursing experience might teach a community health nursing course, and clinical faculty with expertise in nursing leadership might teach the nursing leadership courses. There almost always is congruence between what you are asked to teach and your personal clinical area of expertise. In very few cases, faculty may be asked to teach a course that they don't have much expertise in if there is a critical shortage of faculty, but that should not be the norm.

A typical workweek for clinical faculty may vary based on their specific role, the program the faculty member teaches in, college needs, and level of expertise. Below is an example of what a typical week for a clinical-track assistant professor might look like:

- Two days for clinical supervision of students at the hospital or simulation lab (eight hours each day)
- Half a day for preparing for lecture and clinical
- Half a day for teaching a didactic course or two (online or in person)
- Half a day for office hours to meet with students and respond to emails (responding to emails is typically every day)
- Half a day for required faculty meetings and other service obligations
- One day for grading course assignments and clinical paperwork
- One day for faculty practice

When considering the transition to academia, there are a multitude of factors to contemplate, including finding the ideal balance between satisfactory income, work hours, and personal time. Sometimes these components may be incompatible when transitioning from the bedside or a clinical role to an academic career. Therefore, take the time to conduct a cost-benefit analysis for what this means for you personally and professionally. Regardless, a career in academia can be rewarding and often presents the best of both worlds for nurses eager to maintain their clinical relevance while contributing to educating the next generations of nurses.

Hourly Income vs. Salaried Income

Working in a position to earn hourly income allows flexibility but often uncertainty in the healthcare arena. Hourly pay in a clinical setting can be dictated by the census, business hours, staffing, and other factors contingent on availability of funds. Typically, hourly pay is distributed on a weekly or biweekly basis. Nonetheless, sometimes people feel more comfortable being in an hourly position in a clinical setting because they feel that they have control over what they make.

For example, someone can choose to work extra shifts for overtime when they need to raise money for a particular expense. There is also more flexibility for having multiple jobs without any restrictions (as we discussed in Chapter 1) if the individual is able to satisfy requirements for both employers. Now, whether this is good over time for your mental and physical well-being and patient safety is another topic altogether.

With salaried positions, as is the case in academia, an amount for service is agreed upon for the year and issued monthly or biweekly. These positions can offer security and benefits that include health insurance, vacation pay, and retirement packages. But a salaried employee may also work more hours than initially planned, creating an imbalance between productivity and hourly compensation. Consider the study by Delello and colleagues (2014) that found that faculty members report working an average of 54.35 hours per week, even though salaried faculty positions in academia assume a 40-hour workweek.

Maintaining Clinical Expertise

Another consideration for transition to an academic role is the ability to maintain clinical expertise. There will likely be significantly less availability to practice in your specialty when you take on a full-time role in academia. For some, this may be a relief; for others, it can pose a dilemma when contemplating how to maintain clinical practice hours for national certification requirements. Make sure that you understand how transitioning to academia might affect opportunities to maintain certain certifications, and have a plan for meeting requirements for recertification.

Part-Time vs. Full-Time Faculty

There are many ways to earn income when entering the world of higher education. When beginning a career in academia, some people prefer to test the waters while others dive straight in. If testing the waters is more your speed, be aware that you will earn considerably less in a part-time or adjunct position than full-time faculty. The same rules apply when calculating your hourly pay.

Teaching part time will allow you the freedom to work full time in a different setting where you would typically earn higher wages. This route offers the opportunity of enjoying student interaction while benefiting from the additional income and maintaining clinical relevance. When teaching part time, the responsibilities are fewer, but there can still be time-intensive tasks involved, such as responding to emails, grading assignments, and clinicals.

When teaching full time, you will absorb more responsibilities but earn more annual income than an adjunct position. You may be offered the opportunity to continue practicing clinically, although this varies by university and college. If you are granted approval to practice clinically at another location, some institutions require you to relinquish a percentage of your external earnings to the institution to use at their discretion. Earning income from external clinical practice may be allowed but can be regulated by the institution in conjunction with state or federal law. Inquire upfront and get details in writing before committing to a position.

Time Is Money

Have you ever calculated the dollar value of your time? Unspoken expectations may come into play when you select an academic position. You will be teaching in some capacity, but how much responsibility you have will be determined by your position. If teaching in an adjunct role, you may be offered a flat rate per course. The flat rate of an adjunct role may be attractive to someone seeking consistent supplemental income without a full-time commitment. Therefore, some faculty members prefer adjunct positions as they allow for flexibility to maintain clinical practice while maximizing earning potential.

To determine whether an adjunct role is a good financial decision, divide your salary by the hours you work during and outside of business hours. Do the hours you spend teaching make the compensation worthwhile? If in an adjunct position, to get the best bang for your buck requires excellent time management skills, organizational skills, self-care, and perseverance. A lack of planning on how you will maximize your efforts for the adjunct position might lead to frustration as the role may begin to encroach on your other responsibilities outside academia. Thus, establish early on how much of your time you will allocate each day to your adjunct position and stick to that plan.

The expectation for full-time faculty is typically very different. If your institution offers tenure, you will be expected to engage in research and other scholarly activities on a regular basis. If your institution does not offer tenure to clinical faculty, there may be a lower expectation for research and scholarship you engage in, or it may even be optional. Rank typically determines the expectation for your research and other obligations at the institution of employment. Full-time faculty members are expected to play an active role in faculty meetings, which can be remote or in person and scheduled on different days. These meetings may last longer than planned, depending on the agenda items—so plan accordingly.

Other time-consuming components include answering emails, returning phone calls, attending meetings, and scheduling office hours to meet with students. Other considerations for your role that you should ask about to accurately plan for other responsibilities include clarifying:

- How many courses you are required to teach and the DOE for your particular clinical role
- Whether you are expected to take a practicum course for your assigned role
- Whether course development and revisions are considered as an integral part of your job or if they are extra responsibilities for which you are compensated separately
- The maximum number of students to be enrolled into each practicum course as well as maximum students you can supervise per semester
- The availability of teaching assistants to help with grading assignments and assisting with test proctoring
- The requirements for meeting with students, number of office hours per week, and whether those meetings have to be in person or virtual, depending on the program

Nonetheless, nursing offers vast opportunities to earn supplemental income. This is no different in the world of academia. Although salary is the standard method of compensation, there are other nonclinical methods of earning income—for example, continuing education teaching, institutional agreements, summer teaching, leadership roles (administrative stipend for taking on a leadership role in your college), and consulting. Always be cognizant of limits on external compensation allowed by your institution if you are a full-time clinical faculty.

Distance to Work

An important aspect that I sometimes see people forget to consider is the distance they live from their desired place of employment. Here are some important questions to ask yourself about distance to work that may help you in deciding on transitioning to academia. Do you currently live near an institution where you are interested in working? If not, how long will you spend commuting each day? That time should be calculated into your workday to determine what amount of compensation will be sufficient. You will need to decide the value of your time. Of course, if you will be teaching in a completely online program, this may not be a consideration.

WHITNEE'S LIFE LESSONS

When I began working in academia, I drove an hour to work and an hour home each day. It was challenging to find my footing because I spent so much time in my week traveling to and from work. I was also working as a four-day clinical instructor at the time while practicing as a nurse practitioner. This meant in-person teaching Tuesday through Friday and practicing on Monday, as it was the only day left during the week. I also thought it would be a bright idea to go back to school and pursue a postdoctoral degree for psychiatric mental health. That really narrowed my availability to be productive in half.

I quickly realized that I could not maintain this pace. I also had financial considerations based on how far I lived from work, including the costs of filling up my standard four-door sedan twice a week and maintaining my vehicle. With the 10-12 hours out of my workweek I spent traveling, the workload, the addition of a clinical practice day, and school, I barely had any personal time left at the end. These obstacles may seem like minute issues, but over time, they compound and may create stress and lead to burnout.

If you factor in similar considerations and find yourself in a situation where your finances and personal life may be compromised, you may need to think about other options. You may be able to carpool with other faculty who live close to you. Considering an institution closer to you, a part-time in-person option, or a remote option might all be alternatives. There are many institutions that offer full-time remote positions. Thus, there are many options to consider that may better accommodate your needs—so don't give up on academia!

What Type of Organizational Environment Do You Prefer?

College cultures differ from campus to campus. Each institution provides its own set of core values, mission, vision, and goals that frame the culture.

College Culture Related to Types of Degrees

Most colleges and universities honor DNPs and PhDs as equally prestigious doctoral degrees. However, a few do not offer tenure track as an opportunity for advancement for those holding DNP degrees. While the debate is still ongoing among proponents and opponents of DNP-prepared faculty being eligible for tenure, DNP programs are proliferating across the United States and other countries. Therefore, an increasing number of DNP-prepared faculty are transitioning into academic roles to fill these critical needs of educating DNP students.

In October 2020, the American Association of Colleges of Nursing (AACN), reported 357 DNP programs nationwide, with another 106 programs in the development stages (AACN, 2020b). DNP faculty are clinical experts with the educational preparation to translate research into practice. They are also trained to conduct quality improvement projects and evidence-based practice and are respected leaders in their fields.

The DNP is considered a terminal degree in nursing and as such, should be equally respected within the academic world. Unfortunately, this doesn't always happen. If you are a clinically focused faculty member, knowing how a particular college of nursing views your type of degree program should be an important consideration for transitioning into an academic role at that institution.

Academia as a High Reliability Organization

In the clinical healthcare world, we often use the term *high reliability organization* (HRO). An HRO strives to avoid errors or accidents by focusing on a specific set of principles that help mitigate errors (Sutcliffe, 2011). Universities can and should be HROs. However, this requires adoption and implementation of principles and policies that are consistently adhered to in order to produce excellent student outcomes.

Safety, quality, and efficiency are the structures employed to promote a high reliability organization. These are all essential qualities for a successful academic unit. Therefore, you need to understand what safeguards your college or institution has put in place to ensure consistently excellent student outcomes.

Another hallmark of high reliability organizations is an environment that promotes reporting of unsafe behaviors without fear of retaliation. Asking about these policies and procedures might be of interest to you, especially those dealing with reporting of student misconduct in the clinical setting and how those types of situations have been handled in the past—for example, the guideline for reporting substance use or misuse among students.

Whether dealing with safety, quality, and efficacy issues related to faculty, staff, or students, promoting a *just culture* is important in ensuring that that all concerned individuals are protected. A culture of pointing fingers and favoritism is counterproductive and often leads to dissatisfied employees. Work culture is frequently taken for granted; you may not think about it until you become unhappy. In fact, the culture of the institution you choose can influence your productivity and career progression. Functioning in a positive workplace culture will increase your chances for upward mobility and will also inform your desire to stay. I recommend that you speak to other clinical faculty about their experiences during your job interview process.

Additionally, you want to investigate whether administrators proactively address negativity, bullying, and other adverse behaviors in the workplace. Inability to do so promotes the negative behaviors that may affect the physical and mental well-being of other faculty and staff. Moreover, when other faculty realize that these behaviors are condoned within the college, they too might engage in the negative behaviors, which only exacerbates the situation. This is a recipe for a bad work environment.

A negative workplace environment can cause low faculty and staff engagement, absenteeism, presenteeism, reduced flexibility, and high turnover rates (Daouk-Öyry et al., 2014; Folger, 2021; Menon & Priyadarshini, 2018). Asking a potential employer what the retention rate is for the department and reasons people have provided for leaving the college is a fair question and should offer some insight into working conditions. We discuss this more in Chapter 8.

Choosing a Collaborative Relationship

Depending on which state you hold licensure in, an advanced practice registered nurse (APRN) may be required to initiate a partnership with a physician through a collaborative agreement. A *collaborative agreement* is a legal document that establishes the rights and responsibilities of each party involved. Not all APRNs are required to have collaboration agreements; some have full practice authority. This is important to consider before taking on a faculty practice assignment that may require alternatives to practice considerations. You may also want to know if the college has experience helping faculty establish new collaborative agreements in case your acceptance of the position might require you to get into a different collaborative agreement.

The Collaborative Agreement

APRNs include certified registered nurse practitioners (CRNPs), clinical nurse specialists (CNSs), certified registered nurse anesthetists (CRNAs), and nurse midwives. Your scope of practice will be determined by the board of nursing in the state where you choose to practice. Each level of nursing has a different scope of practice as it pertains to national certification requirements, practice authority, and practice standards.

Collaborative agreements are only utilized when required by the state board of nursing. The collaborative agreement cites the obligation of the collaborating/supervising physician in working with the APRN. In states that celebrate full practice authority, a collaborating agreement is not executed. This means that the APRN is permitted to implement care to the full extent of their scope of practice. If the APRN works for a company other than their own private practice, they may be presented with a contract instead of a collaborating agreement that provides the guidelines and expectations of their role/job description (CRNA, CRNP, CNS, and nurse midwives).

This would be similar to a collaborating agreement minus the third party. For those who work in states that require collaborating agreements, some benefits of this agreement include:

- Having a designated party to reference for consultations and treatment plans and to exchange medical advice
- Offering the patient two providers implementing treatment

However, although the collaborating agreement is meant to guide the working relationship, each provider is individually responsible for the care that is provided to each patient. I recommend that each provider has their own malpractice insurance in place. You may also want to find out if your college offers reimbursement for recertification costs and other faculty practice costs such as malpractice insurance.

Factors to Consider When Choosing a Collaborative Relationship

It is imperative that you research the physician whom you are considering for a collaborative relationship. Ensure that the provider has an unencumbered license and that you can establish a complementary and professional working relationship. Some will charge a fee for collaborating, but this is not a requirement. Make certain that both you and the physician understand your scope of practice.

Furthermore, be prepared to educate physicians about your role and how you can be an asset to their practice. Proactively asking about expectations for workflow and having a clear understanding of the job description will serve you well in the long run. Once you have established the collaborative agreement, schedule regular meetings in advance to review charts, discuss quality assurance, and receive clinical feedback.

APRNs and collaborating physicians do not always work in the same facility. Be clear about the expectations you have or the need for guidance in practice. Establish how you will contact the collaborator when in need of clarification as well as in emergency situations. It is also helpful to have the terms discussed in writing. When establishing a collaboration, a contract may or may not be implemented. This can be an advantage and a disadvantage.

Having an agreement with outlined expectations, contract length, compensation elements, and mutual assents can offer clarity and security. However, this can also impose limitations to your ability to practice, such as limiting your ability to work in other specialties, the geographic location of your practice, and your ability to moonlight. These are consequential components to consider when establishing any collaboration.

Special Consideration for CRNAs

For certified registered nurse anesthetists (CRNAs), the National Board of Certification and Recertification for Nurse Anesthetists (NBCRNA) is the certifying body, and the American Association of Nurse Anesthesiology (AANA) provides the guidelines. The certifying body determines whether or not to grant the approval of continuing education submitted.

> TIPS FOR NEGOTIATING A COLLABORATIVE AGREEMENT
> - Ask clarification questions when ambiguity is present.
> - Restructure how you approach your request, and provide supporting evidence on why your request is reasonable.
> - Provide evidence, company policy, board of nursing guidelines, certification documentation, and any other supporting data that will affirm your expertise.
> - Counter with how you would ultimately like the contract to read.
> - Seek legal counsel to review any contract before endorsing the agreement. This will ensure your best interest is being considered as large institutions generally have a sizable legal team that reviews contracts to protect the sole interest of the institution.

Although no collaboration agreement is needed, some institutions may limit billing options for CRNAs. Thus, if you are a CRNA wishing to transition into an academic role, your practice needs might be slightly different. Make sure you talk to someone who has successfully transitioned to the type of position you are interested in to ensure that you understand these complexities.

Negotiating Your Faculty Clinical Practice

The art of negotiation is not to be taken lightly when discussing your clinical practice time. Take into consideration the workload that will be required when you are working externally. As you negotiate with your potential employer concerning ability to maintain clinical practice while working for the institution, take into consideration all the duties and responsibilities that come with your clinical practice. For example, you may be responsible for your own billing and coding, which may take more than the one day of approved practice time. This will all be determined by the type of facility, the role, and the certification held by the individual.

Negotiating your clinical practice in academia can be overwhelming if you are not sure what the standard is. This is why doing your research and asking the right questions are key. When navigating your way through this tangled web, start by asking yourself:

- What part of my clinical practice brings me the most joy?
- What part of my practice do I enjoy the least?
- What part of my practice is critical to satisfaction?
- What are the requirements to maintain my licensure?

Identify Your Non-Negotiables

When discussing what you want with a potential employer, be upfront about your non-negotiables. If you are currently working every Wednesday with an established clinical partner and want to continue that arrangement, request that upfront. Ask for the agreement in writing, and be sure to inquire if any earnings from external compensation will be withheld by the institution.

If you are holding a full-time appointment, a minimum of one day a week is typically designated for clinical practice. This is the equivalent of one research day a week for tenure-track faculty.

Remote clinical work is also an option to consider when selecting a faculty practice. This option may be more readily available and convenient for your schedule. There are a variety of positions that could be of interest to RNs, CNSs, CRNPs, and CRNAs.

Next, ask about whether the institution has a faculty practice committee. Usually, the purpose of a faculty practice committee is to support faculty who hold formal clinical practices; advocate for issues pertaining to their well-being, including promotion and tenure (if applicable); and provide community and mentorship as needed. The presence of such a committee might be an indication of the attention the college provides to clinical faculty.

Consider the Workload Specific to Your Clinical Practice Role

Not all clinical practice nursing jobs have the same responsibilities or scope of practice. Working on an inpatient unit as a bedside nurse can be extremely taxing on your body, but once you clock out, your responsibility is left at the door. When employed as a case manager, the work may follow you home.

This can be true in an advanced practice position as well. Returning patient calls, following up on prescriptions and refill requests, reviewing requested health information, and charting are tasks that may need to be completed after hours. These responsibilities may not be taken into consideration by leadership when workload credits are issued. Know your boundaries, know your capacity limits, and speak up if you need any accommodations. Asking for a meeting to go over expectations and review the workload assignment is appropriate to ensure a balanced plan for productivity and maintenance of work-life balance.

When negotiating your clinical practice, keep in mind that most of the time the contract is set up to benefit the employer. If there are specific things that you are requesting or there are items that you are considering a need or a want, ask for those things. You might be told no, but that is part of negotiating. Lastly, be on the lookout for clauses that do not align with your plan for self-actualization.

Core Competencies

Core competency is the ability to execute or implement a set of skills required in a particular work setting. These skill sets will differ based on the level of care you are certified to provide. A set of core competencies that all healthcare providers should abide by include professionalism, leadership, communication, knowledge, and business skills.

Each area of specialty has a different set of competencies. For example, the competencies below are created to ensure that nurse practitioners are able to critically analyze data and integrate knowledge while translating it into research (National Organization of Nurse Practitioner Faculties, 2012):

- Scientific foundations
- Leadership
- Quality

- Practice inquiry
- Technology and information literacy
- Policy
- Health-delivery system
- Ethics competencies
- Independent practice competencies

Core competencies for the advanced practice nurse include:

- Direct clinical practice
- Guidance and coaching
- Consultation
- Evidence-based practice
- Leadership
- Collaboration
- Ethical decision-making

These core competencies are factored into the framework of advanced practice development. Hamric's integrated model of advanced practice identifies the role and function of advanced practice nursing (Hamric et al., 2013). Hamric's model (see Figure 7.1) articulates the expectations overall and improves outcomes in healthcare. When considering an academic position, ensure that the position will not inhibit your ability to maintain your core competencies, as that may pose a challenge for recertification.

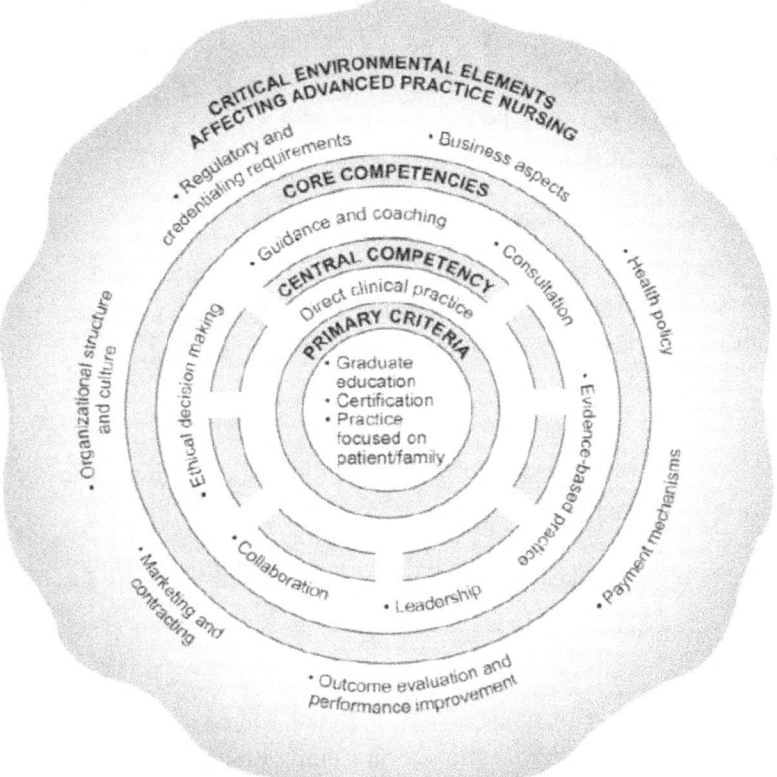

Figure 7.1 Hamric's Integrated Model of Advanced Practice (Tracy & O'Grady, 2017). Reprinted with permission.

Specialty Considerations

One of the reasons nursing is such an exciting career field is the variety of specialties nurses can choose from. Each advanced nursing role has a different scope of practice. If a collaborating provider is required in your state, make sure the provider follows protocol required by their certifying body. Some states require the advanced practice nurse to practice only under the specialty of the collaborating provider. This can be a limiting factor, depending on the geographic location. If you are considering an academic position in a different state, ensure you understand the practice requirements in that state as they may be limiting factors to your ability to take that position.

For example, in rural areas, there may be a limited number of physicians within the specialty available to collaborate with the advanced practice nurse. Other considerations include:

- Board certification hourly requirements for renewal
- Governing body approval for continuing education credits
- DEA license requirements
- Billing and coding regulations
- Financial reimbursement

If you hold more than one certification, you will be responsible for maintaining those certifications. Some employers provide assistance with credentialing and may reimburse you for the time-consuming task. My advice is that that you keep a portfolio of your licensure requirements for renewal, including renewal dates.

WHITNEE'S LIFE LESSONS

When I began my career in academia, I worked each week as a hospitalist NP in my faculty practice position. This role permitted me to leave most of my clinical responsibilities behind when my call shift was over and granted me the flexibility to decompress when leaving work. However, as with many jobs in healthcare, follow-up tasks required additional attention after hours. Other people on my team took care of billing, case management, receptionist duties, and other responsibilities. This reduced the amount of follow-up work I had to do after hours, such as FMLA paperwork, pharmacy phone calls, dictation discrepancies, and other time-consuming tasks. Having a great team is a luxury.

However, small businesses and private practices do not always have the luxury of employing a large team, and that can significantly impact your academic job responsibilities. Make sure that you explain the responsibilities included in your clinical role to your administrators when negotiating your clinical time. Your administrator may not be an APRN, and they may not understand all the nuances of your faculty clinical practice. Having open and honest conversations with your supervising administrator will be beneficial in ensuring that you are not overcommitting to any one aspect of your job, thereby setting you up for success in your clinical faculty position.

Furthermore, before taking on a clinical role, take the time to investigate whether that institution requires you to relinquish part or all of your earnings from your faculty practice to the institution of employment. This may be a deal-breaker for people who are considering academia as an option. Discuss this possibility in-depth with the employer before taking the position.

After I completed my DNP, I was asked to interview for a teaching position. I remember being excited but worried because I thought I would have to choose between clinical practice and higher education. This area was very new to me yet very exciting, and I experienced an internal tug of war. I told myself before I went to the interview that I had worked hard for the opportunity. I was pleased when I learned that a clinical practice day would be granted.

But like many people I have talked to, I forgot to ask about whether the expectation was that part of my earnings from the faculty practice would be remitted to the academic institution. Shortly after taking the position, I learned that funds were being deducted from those who participated in the faculty practice initiative. It is no secret that academia offers less competitive salaries than hospitals, so every penny counted. Since then, I have made sure to encourage other colleagues and friends considering academia to ensure that they ask about this possibility so they can make informed decisions.

Engaging in Research and Scholarship as a Clinical Faculty

If you enter academia as a clinical-track assistant professor, you will be expected to engage in research and scholarly activities. The quantity and frequency of production will be dictated by your rank, contract negotiations, and research ranking for your institution. If you are hired at a research-intensive institution (R01), the expectation to produce excellence and innovation in research on a continual basis is greater compared to a college or university that is less focused on research.

In Chapter 1, we discussed the concept of DOE. The quantity of research and scholarly activity will be dictated by your DOE as well. Your institution should provide benchmarks and guidelines for minimum expectations for promotion and annual merit evaluations. It is your duty to know all applicable policies and procedures.

Steps for Choosing Your Area of Research and Scholarship

Your personal trajectory and passion should guide your research interests. Additionally, your clinical expertise can inform your area of research. Whatever you do, stay focused and intentionally develop a program of research and scholarship that enriches your clinical practice and student experiences. If there is a dean of research in your college, make sure you meet with them and discuss your research and scholarship needs and how your clinical expertise can enrich the projects of other researchers within your college.

Your dean of research can help you make the necessary connections with other researchers within your college or even outside your college. Constructing your scholarship agenda early in your academic career is key to helping you prepare for promotion and your annual merit evaluations. If you aren't sure where to begin, these steps will help:

1. Identify what you are passionate about. Make a list of topics you like to write about, learn more about, and read more about. For example: Do you want to write about suicide rates, organ donation, or cultural competency? Do you want to

learn more about telehealth or cardiovascular disparities? Do you enjoy reading about nursing leadership?

2. Determine the population of your interest. Do you enjoy working with children, patients with disabilities, oncology patients, or patients with mental health issues? It is helpful to assess how much access you will have to the population you select. Think about this in advance if you choose to conduct any human subjects research.

3. Determine what related topics you would like to investigate—for example, health policy, mindfulness, wellness, education, mentoring, pregnancy, or prostate cancer survivors.

4. Add a subset of your choice—for example, gender, age, geography, use of therapy, or use of technology. When in doubt, allow the literature to guide you. I encourage you to write about topics that are exciting for you. This will help reduce the risk of burnout and promote collaboration among your peers and other colleagues.

Observe Your Community

Engaging with the community around you can offer tons of research and scholarship ideas as well as foster a relationship of trust. Research and scholarship ideas may be sitting right in front of you. For example, you may notice that the people in a small, rural community have minimal access to medical care and even less access to mental health services. Raising awareness of alternative methods to seek treatment and planning a health fair for the community could have a life-changing impact on some people. Through these activities, individuals living in these communities may share how they are affected and provide direction for further research. This is the heart of community-engaged research.

Also strive to engage in other forms of scholarly activities as soon as possible. These may include grant writing, conference presentations, and publication of manuscripts. You can also develop CEU events that relate to your clinical expertise and offer them to your colleagues at the college or other individuals in the community. Present your plan for progress and speak with others about their research interest to gauge the possibility of collaborating. The more scholarly activities you engage in, the more prepared you will be for promotion and tenure—if your institution honors your degree as a qualifying factor for tenure track.

Applying for Promotion

Before you commit to an institution as faculty, it is immensely important that you examine your vision for upward mobility. Regardless of whether you are clinical-track or tenure-track faculty, you need to understand the appointment and promotion guidelines for your college. Being knowledgeable about policies will get you on the right track when you first transition into your academic position.

Your department will evaluate your teaching performance, research, scholarship, academic citizenship, and professional contributions. You may also be evaluated on:

- Clinical teaching expertise and consistency of scholarship productivity
- Leadership and professional recognition as well as your engagement in clinical practice
- Teaching innovation. Bringing your clinical practice to the classroom creates critical thinking opportunities that students can easily relate to. Institutions highly value innovative teaching.

- Student and peer evaluations. These will be factored in for consideration of promotion but may have a different weight distribution, depending on the institution.

When working toward promotion, choose quality over quantity, although quantity also matters. Remember that not all opportunities are created equal. Some projects that are a labor of love may not yield recognition equal to other activities based on established criteria. So, while it is important to engage in activities you are simply passionate about, make certain that you are making deliberate efforts to engage in activities that are necessary for promotion and tenure (if applicable). Therefore, work smarter, not harder.

The promotion process, although guided by policy and procedure, may sometimes feel subjective, and applying for promotion can be a tedious, frustrating, and exhausting experience. The antidote for this is keeping up with all aspects of what your organization considers for promotion. Developing a system of organizing your documents will serve you well in the long run.

I encourage new faculty to create a folder called "promotion" on their chosen storage platform. Create subfolders that correspond to each evaluation criterion (e.g., research and scholarship, teaching, service, and professional status). Every time you achieve something related to any of these areas, save the documentation in these folders. For example, if you receive a certificate of attendance for a conference, save that certificate in your professional status subfolder for easy retrieval whenever needed.

While eligibility requirements for promotion and tenure vary, the expectations and guidelines are generally available to internal candidates and interested faculty candidates if they are willing to ask. Understanding rank and the contributions that you will be evaluated on will assist you in documenting your performance and clinical competencies at the desired level for promotion.

Depending on the culture of the institution, which scholarly activities may or may not count toward this evaluation process may differ. Before going up for promotion, ensure that you request an internal review to gauge how you are doing. This is especially important if there is not a requirement to have your dossier evaluated annually for promotion as clinical faculty (as is the case for tenure-track faculty). Lastly, be sure to ask for clarification on both quality and quantity of your body of work during the internal review process before you officially go up for promotion and tenure (if applicable). This will prevent you from having any surprises when you submit your final dossier.

Final Thoughts

Clinical faculty are valuable members of colleges of nursing. They bring with them a vast array of experiences and expertise that are essential to the preparation of students for clinical practice, leadership, and community service. Nonetheless, it is important to understand what your clinical role entails. This chapter includes a thorough discussion of the various aspects of being a clinical faculty—strategies to be successful as well as pitfalls to avoid. You can thrive and flourish in academia as a clinical faculty. You have what it takes!

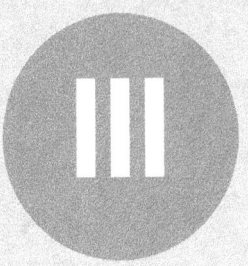

III

IT STARTS AND ENDS WITH YOU: MIND, BODY, AND SOUL

8   Othering in Academia: An Imperative for
    Diversity, Equity, and Inclusion 169

9   Stress Management 101 205

10 Thriving in Academia 223

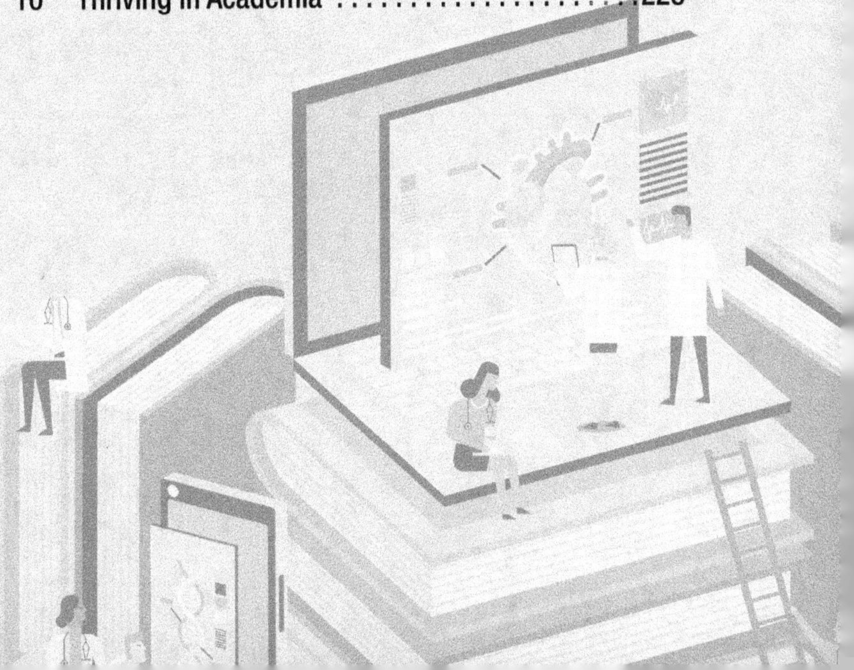

8

OTHERING IN ACADEMIA: AN IMPERATIVE FOR DIVERSITY, EQUITY, AND INCLUSION

I thought long and hard about including a chapter on racial equity and inclusion in this book because of the sensitive nature of the topic. I initially opted to only address the issue as a subsection related to my personal experience, but I'm glad that my editors encouraged me to dedicate a chapter to this topic.

This chapter is not an indictment of the nursing profession or of academia. I love being a nurse and an academic—but it is imperative that we have open and honest conversations about othering in nursing and in academia. This is an issue that people do not readily talk about, but it has far-reaching implications for many individuals. Please do not have any trepidation or feel like you need to put on armor as if we are going to war; my hope is that by learning about the factors that contribute to systemic racism, we will be equipped to recognize it and will have strategies and skillsets that allow all of us to be part of the solution.

To provide a multifaceted discussion of othering in academia, a few friends and colleagues who are white contributed their personal experiences and perspectives, which add a certain richness to our conversation. The diversity of perspectives educates all of us by showing that we are more alike than different, and if we choose to focus on the things that truly matter, we can achieve more as a profession.

Defining Othering

Kathryn Minshew says that "a company is only as good as its people. The hard part is actually building the team that will embody your company culture and propel you forward" (Minshew, as cited in Zsurzsan, 2014, para. 7). In the same vein, I say that an organization is only as healthy as its employees (physically, mentally, psychosocially, etc.). On the surface, it may look like the organization is thriving. But if some members of the organization are suffocating because of inequities and inequalities they experience on a regular basis, eventually the organization will stagnate or crumble—whether metaphorically or literally.

Othering is a complex construct that has been defined in several ways. The Macmillan Dictionary (n.d., para. 1) defines *othering* as "treating people from another group as essentially different from and generally inferior to the group you belong to."

Based on this definition, it is not necessarily recognizing differences among groups that poses the most harm, but rather the belief that people who are different from you are generally inferior. Therefore, although it used to be a socially acceptable statement for people to say they are "color blind," we now know that this is inadequate—it is necessary to dig deeper into the historical and social context of racial inequities.

Not doing so stymies the necessary growth and development required to recognize and address the deep-seated prejudices and assumptions (conscious or subconscious) that we may have. These prejudices and assumptions inform individual belief systems that ultimately manifest as bias, discrimination, or racism. Therefore, there is nothing wrong with acknowledging that human beings are uniquely created and can be different in many ways—as long as different does not equal inferior.

Clint Curle (n.d.), a human rights researcher, explains that:

> People are different. We can use our differences as an opportunity to share and learn or we can use our differences as an excuse to build walls between us. When we highlight differences between groups of people to increase suspicion of them, to insult them or to exclude them, we are going down a path known as "othering." (para. 1)

Thus, the problem with othering is that it creates a framework through which systemic and structural inequalities are justified and perpetuated. Moreover, understanding its origins and manifestations is foundational to developing and implementing strategies that counteract the deleterious effects of othering in our society. To achieve this, a deliberate and collective awakening of the consciousness that stands up to injustice and promotes equity at all levels is required. This may seem like an arduous task to take on, but in the words of Nelson Mandela, one of the world's most influential leaders: "It always seems impossible until it's done."

A Historical Perspective on Othering

Our global society has a long history of othering. Unfortunately, that centuries-long history includes tragedies and human rights violations such as the Holocaust, transatlantic slave trade, Rwandan Genocide, displacement of Native Americans in North America, Haiti Massacre, ethnic cleansing of Circassia, apartheid, and many more. Othering is a global problem that has indiscriminately plagued various societies for centuries.

The danger of othering is that it does not always culminate into large-scale, horrific events—it can have subtle consequences that can be easily overlooked by society at large. This often results in the systematic silencing of the oppressed who may want to speak up against the ills perpetrated against them. The idea that if an issue does not affect the majority of the people, then it is not an issue worth addressing is what leads those who choose to speak up against inequalities and inequities to be targeted and labeled as the problem. Consequently, an unhealthy environment of us-versus-them is created—and designed—to keep the status quo and prevent change at all costs, even if it means that organizational outcomes suffer.

> *"No matter how big a nation is, it is no stronger than its weakest people, and as long as you keep a person down, some part of you has to be down there to hold him down, so it means you cannot soar as you might otherwise."*
>
> *–Marian Anderson*

Othering in Academia

The academic environment possesses many of the conditions in which othering can thrive. From power dynamics to the politics of governance and to the intersectionality of race and gender—all these conditions have been shown to contribute to othering in society and specifically in academia. In Chapters 1 and 2, we discussed understanding formal and informal hierarchies in academia and their impact on professional growth and development. However, when you are a faculty member from a minority group, there are additional complexities to consider as you contemplate transitioning into an academic role.

For example, in a 2013 study by British Black faculty that examined racial equity in academia, 56% of respondents identifying as Black or from an ethnic minority group reported discrimination, and 73% indicated that their institution's performance in promoting equity was either poor or very poor. This study also found that Black or ethnic minority faculty felt that they were not taken seriously and had numerous experiences with racism and contemptuous treatment (Parr, 2014).

The factors that contribute to these experiences for Black and minority faculty are many and varied. Nonetheless, the evidence is clear and well documented. The experiences of Black and other minority faculty as a result of unfair practices either set them up for failure or are intended to create a hostile environment that forces them to leave academia without realizing their highest potential. Such practices may include lack of mentoring and role modeling, different performance expectations, lack of leadership opportunities, overt and covert bias and discrimination, blatant disrespect, unequal pay, and minimizing or devaluing of Black faculty's personal achievements (Hassouneh et al., 2014; Pololi et al., 2010; Pololi et al., 2013).

It is pivotal as a Black or minority faculty that you explore your institution's policies and procedures related to diversity, equity, and inclusion prior to accepting a position at that institution. I previously mentioned that it is very helpful to consider having meetings and discussions with Black or minority faculty at that institution to explore their experiences as employees. Depending on the environment at the institution (e.g., history of retaliation), you may or may not get an honest answer. At a minimum, you will be able to decipher from the answers presented, the enthusiasm with which the topic is discussed, and perhaps even the body language whether minority faculty are genuinely happy at that institution. I always advise people to pay closer attention to nonverbal cues when discussing this issue than what is actually said.

In 2021, several incidences of Black and minority faculty pushing back on the establishment and confronting racism in academia were reported (Anderson, 2021). These stories represent only a handful of the discriminatory systems and practices that Black and other minority faculty experience consistently in academia. According to Hassouneh et al. (2014), these practices are achieved through systemic and structural patterns of exclusion and control, which consequently force Black and minority faculty into a perpetual state of surviving with occasional breakthroughs of thriving. Thus, for many Black and minority faculty, the ability to survive and ultimately thrive is dependent on the severity of the exclusion and control and access to mentorship. Later in this chapter, we talk more about the importance of a minority faculty having a mentor from a minority background.

Hassouneh et al. (2014) further state that patterns of exclusion and control happen through three main "simultaneous, interrelated, and mutually reinforcing sub-processes" (para. 20): the invalidation of a sense of self, the establishment of unequal standards and access to resources, and othering. Invalidation of the sense of self occurs when individual strengths and characteristics of faculty of color are strategically ignored and are replaced with ongoing personal assaults that have no bearing on the professional knowledge possessed by the faculty member.

For example, faculty from a dominant group may choose to focus on the personal style of a Black professor and attack that image as "unprofessional," while intentionally ignoring all the professional achievements and recognition the faculty member brings to the institution through their teaching, scholarship, and service. This practice intentionally dehumanizes the individual and leads to stereotyping based on negative group characteristics to justify the discriminatory practices being implemented.

Similarly, establishment of unequal standards and access to resources disadvantages minority faculty by limiting their ability to succeed at the same level compared to their white counterparts. This double standard creates disparities in performance that inadvertently portray minority faculty as underperformers compared to their white counterparts. For example, the literature shows that minority faculty receive significantly higher teaching loads, receive poorer performance reviews, and are less likely to be promoted (Abelson et al., 2018; Crayton, 2019; Peterson et al., 2004).

This double standard also creates an atmosphere in which minority faculty cannot afford to be average. They seemingly have to outperform their white counterparts to receive the same and sometimes even less recognition or promotion, which maintains the state of survival for Black and minority faculty. Consequently, minority faculty may exhibit poor mental health (depression, stress, and anxiety) and physical health outcomes. Unequal standards can also contribute to imposter syndrome of Black and minority faculty. These factors combined often result in the faculty member leaving an institution because of feelings of helplessness (Zamudio-Suarez, 2021).

> **SUCCESS NUGGET**
>
> Unfortunately, race-related double standard is a frequently occurring phenomenon, and in organizational cultures where it persists, the turnover rate of Black and minority faculty is often high. If you are a person from a minority group and are thinking about transitioning into an academic role, it is important for you to research retention rates for minority faculty at your institution. It might also be helpful to compare average length of employment for Black and minority faculty compared to white faculty. This might be a good indicator of the experiences of Black faculty at your institution and a proxy for job satisfaction.

Intersectionality of Race and Gender

Although our discussion in this chapter focuses on racial and ethnic minorities, othering is often experienced by many individuals from other marginalized groups, including sexual and gender minorities

(SGM). Understanding the intersectionality of identities in academia and the corresponding compounded effects of othering in this subset of individuals is equally important. Additional supports and resources are essential in mitigating the impacts of othering in these populations. This is particularly important in academia, where a historically patriarchal, white, and heterosexual male hierarchy has been maintained for centuries (Ajil & Blount-Hill, 2020; Phiri, 2018).

Disparities related to women in general and minority women in particular are staggering. For instance, although the majority of non-tenure lecturers are women, women make up only 44% of tenure-track faculty, 36% of full professors, and 30% of college presidents. Additionally, female faculty members still make less than their male counterparts with comparable experience at every academic rank. Interestingly, only 5% of college presidents identify as female and a member of a racial or ethnic minority group (American Association of University Women, n.d.; Bichsel & McChesney, 2017).

Although nurses are predominantly female, understanding these issues is critical as colleges of nursing do not operate in silos. Nursing faculty must be aware of these dynamics and disparities as they collaborate with colleagues from other colleges or academic units. This is especially true for women of color. To counteract these effects, McKinsey & Company (2021) recommends implementation of allyship to support women of color in the workplace. We delve into allyship later in this chapter.

> *"No country can ever truly flourish if it stifles the potential of its women and deprives itself of the contributions of half of its citizens."*
>
> –Michelle Obama

Race and Racism in Nursing

When I first started nursing school, I began hearing that "nurses eat their young." The more I learned what this meant, the more disturbing the phrase became to me. In a caring profession that has consistently been ranked as the most trusted profession for 20 consecutive years (Saad, 2022), I just couldn't fathom how it was possible for nurses to eat their young. The same was true as I started learning about race and experiencing racism in nursing.

Earlier in the book, I mentioned that I was born and raised in Zambia, Africa. When I was growing up, I never experienced racism, and in fact, people who looked like me were the majority. I often kid and say that I actually did not realize that I was Black until I moved to the United States. For 18 years of my life, I thought I was just a human being. And for the first time in my life, I was forced to check a box and identify with a certain group—I was instantly boxed into certain stereotypical expectations for what was possible for "someone who looks like me."

As I've talked to several Black and minority nurses over the years, I've learned that experiences of racism are not unique to me. Furthermore, the literature clearly shows that we have a problem in nursing that transcends area of practice—from acute care to long term care, from academia to industry, and from community-based nursing to executive leadership (National Commission to Address Racism in Nursing, 2021). We have to do something about this issue, and we have to do it now.

Black nurses consistently report feeling professionally invisible and cannot find legitimate reasons for their inability to advance professionally (Wilson, 2007). Additionally, fewer Black nurses advance into leadership positions, pursue doctoral degrees, or transition into academic roles, which inadvertently negatively impacts minority students because they do not have enough role models to inspire them to pursue desired career trajectories (Brinkert, 2010; Cortisman, 2008).

Black faculty often report patterns of communication by their white colleagues that are perceived as racist (Robinson, 2013). Moreover, Black faculty often fear being poorly evaluated by their students when they bring up issues of race in the classroom (Hassouneh, 2006). Lastly, Black nursing students also report that white students are uncomfortable talking about race and racism (Sue et al., 2009). Sometimes nonverbal cues of disagreements such as rolling of eyes and avoiding eye contact are exhibited. Similarly, when student discussions about race and racism arise, Black students have reported unhelpful responses from their teachers, who dismiss the issues raised as unimportant or expect racial minority students to be experts on topics of race and racism (Hall & Fields, 2012).

Manifestations of Othering and Racism

There are three major factors that contribute to the systemic perpetuation of othering and racism in academic (and other) institutions.

Bias

Bias is "a tendency to believe that some people, ideas, etc., are better than others that usually results in treating some people unfairly" (Merriam-Webster, n.d.-a, para. 1). There are different types of biases, including confirmation bias, affinity bias, priming, anchoring bias, and value attribution. Work in this area has also been expanded to address *implicit bias*, which is the area we will be focusing on for the purposes of this discussion. But first, below are a few types of biases and their definitions (Burton-Hughes, 2017):

- *Confirmation bias* is the tendency to look for facts that support our ideas or beliefs about certain issues.
- *Affinity bias* happens when we prefer to associate with people who have similar values as this makes us feel safe and relatable.

- *Priming* refers to phenomenon whereby previous experiences or stimuli prime/influence how one unintentionally or unconsciously responds to other stimuli in the future.
- *Anchoring bias* is the tendency to rely more heavily on information that was first available to us, whereby any new information is seen through the lens of the initial information, thereby decreasing objectivity.
- *Value attribution* refers to how we perceive our actions and those of others by assigning them to a particular outcome.

Early work on implicit bias was birthed out of the realization that many people have biases or even covert prejudices that are outside the realm of their consciousness (Greenwald et al., 1998). It is important for all of us to be aware of our implicit biases because they usually precipitate the establishment of unequal standards and inequitable allocation of resources among minority groups. This bias systematically disadvantages individuals who identify with these groups.

It is important to note that we all have biases. The solution is to be aware of our biases and to ensure that they do not inform how we treat people who are different from us. These realizations are critical for nursing because our work extends beyond how we treat each other to how we treat our patients. Addressing implicit bias has the potential to close health equity gaps and improve population outcomes. Faculty need to recognize bias (implicit or explicit) to know when to advocate for themselves or others.

A study by Joseph and Davis (2021) explored whether nursing students are aware of their implicit biases and how they affect their care of individuals from different races and backgrounds. The study found that 80% of student participants were previously not exposed to the concept of implicit bias; they openly acknowledged that how they were raised significantly contributed to their biases and believed that implicit biases affect the quality and equity of care provided to their patients. Similar results were found among practicing nurses, except that in this sample, implicit biases did not impact clinical decision-making (Haider et al., 2015).

Strategies to Combat Implicit Bias

The good news is that biases can be mitigated. Edgoose et al. (2019) propose eight strategies to combat implicit bias:

- Introspection
- Mindfulness practice
- Perspective-taking
- Slowing down
- Individuation
- Checking one's messaging
- Institutionalizing fairness
- Take two

Introspection

Introspection allows each of us to examine our own values, belief systems, and prejudices and how they influence how we treat people from groups that are different from us. Edgoose et al. (2019) also suggest completing implicit bias tests so we can have objective data that might inform our actions to combat implicit bias.

Mindfulness Practice

Practicing mindfulness allows us to be present in a moment in a nonjudgmental context, which can reduce stress and improve self-awareness. Being present in the moment also allows us to only use the information available and within the situated context, which then improves objectivity.

Perspective-Taking

We often refer to perspective-taking as being in someone else's shoes. Oftentimes, when we take the time to understand how the implicit bias negatively affects the stereotyped individual, we are more likely to be empathetic and change behavior accordingly.

Slowing Down

Learning to slow down allows us time to evaluate our biases before interacting with others, thereby diminishing reflexive reactions. This strategy can also help us to be kinder and more considerate in our interactions with other people.

Individuation

Individuation is the process by which people develop unique characteristics that differentiate them from others in society or from a similar group (Merriam-Webster, n.d.-b). In this context, individuation requires that we treat people based on their personal characteristics instead of assigning values based on the groups to which they may be affiliated. This prevents stereotyping and, ultimately, othering.

Checking One's Messaging

Checking one's messaging is important because sometimes we are not even aware of how our actions are being perceived by others. Additionally, taking the time to learn evidence-based language and embracing multiculturism may minimize implicit bias.

Institutionalizing Fairness

Institutionalizing fairness is one of the most important strategies to combat implicit bias in the workplace because it promotes equity in all aspects of organizational operation. When an organization embraces a culture of fairness and does not tolerate discrimination, employees are more likely to address their own biases.

Take Two

Take two is a concept that requires practicing cultural humility and engagement in lifelong learning that produces self-awareness. We'll talk more about cultural humility when we discuss antidotes for othering and racism.

Microaggressions

The term microaggression was first coined in 1978 by Chester Pierce, an African American Professor and psychiatrist at Harvard. He defined *microaggressions* as "subtle, stunning, often automatic, and nonverbal exchanges which are 'putdowns'" (Pierce et al., 1978, p. 66). This definition has since been expounded to the idea that microaggressions cause harm to the target, whether intentionally or unintentionally, and are not just "putdowns" (Sue, 2010). According to Sue and Spanierman (2020), microaggressions represent the complex interaction of microinteractions and macrostructures, which manifest as systemic inequities at the societal level.

Therefore, while occasional microaggressions may be harmless, the long-term subjugation to such experiences can have detrimental effects. It is also important to note that the microinteractions are happening within the context of macrosystems that often provide the environments and conditions in which these microaggressions proliferate. Sue (2010) and Sue et al. (2007) have classified microaggressions into microassaults, microinsults, and microinvalidations.

- *Microassault* is "an explicit racial derogation characterized primarily by a verbal or nonverbal attack meant to hurt the intended victim through name-calling, avoidant behavior, or purposeful discriminatory actions" (Sue et al., 2007, p. 274).

- *Microinsult* comprises rudeness and insults that are conveyed through everyday conversations and are intended to demean the cultural heritage of the targeted person.

- *Microinvalidation* comprises communications that is often unconscious that is intended to exclude, invalidate, or nullify a person's thoughts or feelings.

As can be seen from these characteristics, microassaults, microinsults, and microinvalidations are not only aimed at attacking the inherent value of the individual—they often lead to denial that othering and racism even exist. These acts also place the burden of proving the discrimination and prejudice on the victim. The mental burden associated with experiencing microaggression can have physiological effects and increase depression, anxiety, and stress—and can even exacerbate imposter syndrome. We talk more about imposter syndrome in Chapter 10.

Therefore, Spanierman et al. (2021) caution against the misrepresentation and underestimation of the dangerous effects of microaggressions as "micro" in nature. The term *micro* is only used to reference the fact that these egregious acts are at the interpersonal level, not necessarily the impact of the actions.

SUCCESS NUGGET

If you are a member of a minority group, I want you to remember that your experiences are valid. I cannot tell you how many times I have heard people question whether they are overthinking an issue or overreacting based on how someone else treated them. I just want you to know that if you do experience these things, you are not going crazy, and you are not overreacting. You need to take steps to identify these issues and engage in healthy strategies to protect yourself and your mental health.

According to Harrison and Tanner (2018), no one solution is effective at addressing microaggressions. Nonetheless, several strategies are provided that might be useful in dealing with microaggressions, whether you are the target or a bystander. These include:

- Acknowledging the microaggression and increasing awareness of potential harms
- Acknowledging the resulting negative feelings and assisting the affected individual by lessening the cognitive load associated with evaluating whether their feelings are valid
- Confronting the microaggression and making sure that the perpetrator understands that this behavior is unacceptable in the workplace
- Making oneself available to and supportive of people experiencing microaggressions
- Meeting with and coaching individuals who are engaging in microaggression to provide an opportunity to correct their behavior without embarrassing them

> *"Prejudice is a burden that confuses the past, threatens the future, and renders the present inaccessible."*
>
> –Maya Angelou

Despite the overwhelming evidence, often I run into colleagues who deny that racism is an issue in nursing. Their reasons for thinking so include:

- They believe they have never personally treated anyone poorly based on the color of their skin or their belonging to a different group.

- The example I provided to describe racism or discrimination is something they personally do not think is a problem or cannot identify with.
- They have never viewed a particular situation as racist or discriminatory and therefore do not consider it a valid example.

To get over this hump, I often suggest a conversation on a somewhat controversial topic—white privilege.

SHIRLEY'S LIFE LESSON

"You cannot dismantle what you cannot see. You cannot challenge what you do not understand."

–Layla F. Saad

Awareness of my own privilege as a white person appears in front of me slowly, like swatches of color from a paintbrush on a large mural. Gradually, the painters create a very different view of the world from what was painted for me by my ancestors. Sometimes I add my own strokes of color as I seek to fill in gaps by doing my own inner work. I realize that I choose to engage with this mural or not; in my white privilege, I have the choice of which world, which reality I will engage in.

No one uttered the term *white privilege* in my presence or wrote about race-related privilege in school textbooks that I read growing up. The term received more attention in the press around the time I graduated from college in 1988, when McIntosh (1989) described both white and male privilege. However, I did not encounter the term until years later.

White privilege was not in my consciousness as a small child. I spent most of my formative years in an all-white, middle-class bubble in Waco and later Arlington, Texas. My relatives held a mix of views on race. I was an eager learner, sitting quietly, listening to the grownups talk around me. They lovingly created the safe white landscape for me. Despite some good examples by individual members, I feel generational shame as I recall comments made and beliefs held by relatives on both sides of my family.

The colorful mural of life emerged for me in elementary school when Waco Independent School District integrated in 1972. I recall playing as equals on the playground with Black children from across town. My third-grade self painted an angry picture of a Black friend who had been a math whiz but stopped performing well in school. I believed that she did not want to stand out from her Black peers. In fourth grade, I watched the television series "Roots" with horror, filling in a large portion of my mental mural.

I spent most of my growing-up years in almost all white schools and churches, never stepping out of my white privilege comfort zone until early adulthood. I added more brush strokes to my life-mural in nursing school and during work as a nurse. Graduate school restructured my worldview, setting the stage for a new level of awareness. There, I learned about social structures that promoted health disparities. Work in academia and later as a nurse scientist has given me opportunities for rich discussions with intelligent minds from diverse walks.

This long-term visual restructuring project causes me anguish as I grapple with awareness of white privilege. I am reexamining deeply held beliefs, looking at beloved family members with fresh eyes, and contemplating my actions. I continue to receive this awareness slowly, across time. I have gained skills along the way that have helped me have compassion for myself and others in this process. Mindfulness meditation practices help me to stay grounded and see my inner thoughts and feelings. Discussions with other nurses and diverse professionals help me grasp a bigger view of the world. Reading fiction and nonfiction works on topics that deal with racism and give voice to persons of color has helped me grow. Through all of this, I have benefited from a practice of self-compassion to cope with the emotional pain of white privilege awareness and sort through appropriate actions. I wonder what this beautiful mural will reveal next.

Understanding White Privilege

The Oxford English Dictionary defines *white privilege* as "inherent advantages possessed by a white person on the basis of their race in a society characterized by racial inequality and injustice" (n.d.-d).

This term sometimes evokes certain defensive emotions and behaviors because it is perceived to imply that the advantages enjoyed by our white colleagues automatically forfeit or diminish their effort, skills, or expertise. But this could not be further from the truth.

In her book *Witnessing Whiteness*, Shelly Tochluk (2010) recounts why conversations about white privilege are inherently difficult. She acknowledges that:

> It is highly disconcerting and offensive to be told that you are unconscious of what influences your attitudes and beliefs about the world. The insinuation that unrecognized socialization was largely responsible for my thinking and actions … but unfortunately, as offensive as an idea might sound, it still may be true. (p. xiii)

In one of the seminal works on white privilege, Peggy McIntosh (1989) provides what I believe is a rationale for extending grace when having conversations about white privilege. According to her, most white people are unconsciously and systematically socialized to deny white privilege. She argues that this intentional denial is reinforced because to accept this reality is to become "newly accountable" (para. 4). And once people are accountable, they must take responsibility for their actions.

The most important conversation to be had regarding privilege is that most of us are socialized to hold certain belief systems without even realizing it. Additionally, none of us can choose the families or societies in which we are born. We just tend to show up, right? Therefore, speaking about privilege should not be perceived as a personal attack. I often encourage people to enter these conversations with grace and not condemnation. In Chapter 8 of her book, Tochluk (2010) provides various strategies that can be utilized to bring people to the table so that these important conversations can take place.

These include:

- Building knowledge about race and racism and their relationship to whiteness through examining one's own life, diversifying informational sources and outlets, and seeking new experiences
- Building skills, including speaking up and naming the problem, practicing responses to racism, and inviting dialogue that centers on diversity
- Building capacity by creating strong and healthy sense of self, depersonalizing appropriately, and appreciating the intimacy that comes with conflict
- Creating a community of people who are purposeful and intentional in their desire to promote racial equity

KRISTEN'S LIFE LESSON

In May 2020, an African nurse whom I work closely with here in the U.S. contacted me. She was deeply troubled by the murder of George Floyd and the events that followed. I asked about her experience with racism in America. At the time, I naively believed that a first-generation African immigrant would have a different experience from an African American. I was shocked by her responses and struck by the absolute vacuum of discrimination I have experienced as a white middle-class woman.

I have never had the experience of a patient taking one look at me and refusing my care. My Black colleagues have this experience regularly and handle it with grace and professionalism. I was deeply troubled to learn that my African friends never experienced racism until they came to this country. When I am among African friends, it rarely occurs to me that I am the only white person there. I am not treated with racism; I am treated as a valued guest.

> I am absolutely guilty of not reflecting on my white privilege, and worse, of not teaching my children. I have long been aware of and troubled by the severe racial disparities in maternal and infant mortality and morbidity, but I hadn't let the profound impact of systemic racism really sink into my understanding. Now I make deliberate efforts to better understand the experience of being Black in America and to share what I learn with my students. My current students are the future of nursing. I want them to understand the impact of privilege and systemic racism sooner than I did. I want them to explore their own attitudes and values around race, to become aware of their own implicit biases, and to go forth and change this country into a place that sees and values every human being.

Although I'm not the friend in Kristen's story, I too have experienced countless incidents where a patient has refused to receive my care because of the color of my skin. Kristen actually has quite a unique background—her mother is white, and her father is Cherokee. She and I have had many conversations about race, discrimination, and privilege. What has facilitated these conversations is open and honest dialogue that is housed in a nonjudgmental and safe environment. We both choose to create that environment with the people we encounter every day.

I encourage all of us to have these conversations because that is where the solutions lie—the wherewithal to develop an inviting and nonthreatening atmosphere in which we can pursue equity collectively and passionately for all human beings. So where do we go from here, and how do we ensure more of such conversations are taking place in our profession? Following is a discussion of the antidotes for othering and racism in academia as well as the profession of nursing.

> *"We rise by lifting others."*
>
> —Robert Ingersoll

The Antidotes for Othering in Academia

The antidotes for othering in academia are multifaceted, multilevel strategies that are aimed not only at dismantling both structural and systemic frameworks (macro level) that have contributed to othering but also individual-level interventions that affect interpersonal outcomes (micro level). These strategies include:

- Increasing diversity in the workforce
- Creating inclusive work environments
- Implementing equitable practices
- Adopting a mindset of cultural humility
- Developing allyship with faculty from minority groups

Increasing Diversity in the Workforce and Among Students

Right now, diversity, equity, and inclusion seem like global buzzwords, but let's move from the superficial application of these concepts toward a more practical and sustainable incorporation at every level of the organizational structures. This vision is in line with the American Association of Colleges of Nursing (AACN; 2021) diversity, equity, and inclusion position statement. To achieve this, AACN identifies three imperatives for academic nursing:

1. Improving the quality of education by promoting learning from individuals representing different life experiences, backgrounds, and perspectives

2. Addressing pervasive health inequalities by ensuring that the nursing workforce can meet the needs of diverse patient populations

3. Enhancing the civic readiness and engagement of nursing students who will be the future leaders of our profession and society

We often say that representation matters. But what does this even mean? Minority faculty are used to being the "first" or "only" in many settings. While this spells progress at many levels, this reality often gives birth to what is now termed the invisible labor of minority faculty (June, 2015; Troung, 2021). This refers to the reality that when minority faculty end up the first or only in different circumstances, there is a commensurate burden to represent one's group well, the pressure to be the voice of the group you identify with, and the unseen weight of mentorship for a significant number of students who may look up to you as a role model for what is possible.

It might seem radical, but Kimberly Truong (2021), the Chief Equity Officer at MGH Institute of Health Professions at Harvard University, actually proposed and implemented, with university support, a reduced workload requirement for faculty of color at her institution that takes into account the invisible labor hours that minority faculty put into supporting students and helping their institutions succeed.

Representation matters among college leadership, faculty, students, and staff to ensure that we are decreasing the invisible labor of faculty of color so that they are not drowning from workload that nonminority faculty may not even know exists. Your institution may not be able to implement such a significant change; however, what we are advocating for is an acknowledgement of this invisible labor and the appropriate readjustment of other duties and responsibilities as necessary.

A PERVASIVE MISCONCEPTION: DIVERSITY DECREASES QUALITY

In my experience, it is not that people don't want to increase diversity in academia or other settings. What I have found is that people have a fear that increasing diversity negatively impacts the quality of the nursing program. For example, I have often heard people ask, "Will we be affecting the quality of the program if we implement the holistic admission process?" And while such statements may be viewed as benign by the faculty from dominant groups, it is actually quite offensive because it insinuates that people of color or minorities (whether students, faculty, or others) are inferior, and their inclusion will result in plummeting of educational standards at that institution.

This perception leads to othering of minority students and unfair grading practices (Fyfe et al., 2022). The unconscious biases and the imputed inferiority of minority students lead to harsher grading so that the faculty member can feel justified in their prejudice when minority students underperform compared to their white counterparts. These practices create a vicious cycle that hinders matriculation and progress of minority students, resulting in high attrition rates estimated at anywhere from 15–85% (Loftin et al., 2012). Additionally, students of color often feel discriminated against by white students who may be socialized to believe that their counterparts from minority groups are not as intelligent as they.

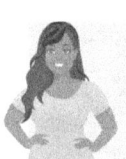

MERCY'S MOMENTS

I remember this like it was yesterday. It was my very first class at the university after I moved to the United States, a U.S. government course. One of the very first assignments in that course was a group assignment. The class was divided into groups of five. We were instructed to meet as a group after class to decide how to divide up the assignment and to establish preliminary due dates for the group. On the first day of class, the professor had asked us to introduce ourselves. Of course, I went on to tell the class that this was my first time in the U.S. and my first college course, but I was excited to be here and to learn.

As we started reintroducing ourselves, one of the girls in the group looked at me and asked, "You are the girl from Africa, right?" I said, "Yes I am. My name is

Mercy." She then said, "Well, I will have to ask the professor how he thinks this will work for our group since we technically only have four people on our team, and other groups have five." At first, it didn't dawn on me what she meant. During the next class period, she asked our professor about it and was told that I counted as a student and would be expected to contribute my fair share.

I was surprised that this girl automatically concluded that I could not positively contribute to the assignment because I was from Africa. But I don't blame her. All she probably knew about Africa were the stories she saw on TV about war-torn areas with children starving to death. And while that may be the case in some parts of Africa, making an assumption about someone before you even have the opportunity to get to know them is why we need exposure to more diverse groups of people at all levels of society.

Representation in academic leadership is equally important. While individuals can make a difference at micro levels, academic leadership buy-in is required to make the type of systemic and structural changes required to promote a culture—and the infrastructure necessary to support the implementation of equitable, inclusive, and accessible environments in which all faculty can thrive. Therefore, the onus is on our academic leaders to commit to this important work and to allocate the necessary resources to ensure sustainability of such environments within the academic setting.

Creating an Inclusive Workplace and Implementing Equitable Practices

The AACN (2021) defines *inclusion* as representing "environmental and organizational cultures in which faculty, students, staff, and administrators with diverse characteristics thrive" (para. 9). It is important to pay attention to the word *thrive* in this definition. Earlier in the chapter, I mentioned that the organization is only as healthy as its members. Therefore, inclusive environments that allow everyone to thrive are fostered through intentional embracing of differing perspectives, experiences, and cultures.

Inclusive environments are facilitated by mutual respect and not simply tolerance of one another. Inclusive workplaces are a byproduct of equitable practices that afford all faculty, staff, and students access to the same resources and supports. This includes equitable pay, teaching assignments, and recognition. Although it is everyone's responsibility to create and uphold inclusive work environments, it really starts from the top; therefore, academic administrators have the responsibility to ensure that minority faculty in their academic units feel valued and acknowledged and are treated as integral parts of the organization.

Creating inclusive workplaces also requires promotion of belonging. Belonging is cultivated through a shared mission and vision as well as through building community, which result in feelings of connectedness. The Center for Creative Leadership (2022) warns against unintended consequences of diversity, equity, and inclusion initiatives when they are not done correctly:

- Tokenism happens when diverse individuals are hired only for the sake of meeting certain quotas without genuine regard for the person. This is a poor approach to increasing diversity because it does not promote true representation. This sentiment is also echoed by Iheduru-Anderson et al. (2022).
- Assimilation happens when individuals from the minority group try to fit into the organizational culture. The danger of assimilation is that it diminishes diversity of thought and perspective and is counterproductive to the heart of true diversity, equity, and inclusion initiatives.
- Dehumanization happens when someone is not treated with the same respect as other members of the team and is made to feel less intelligent or capable compared to their colleagues from the dominant group.

Academic leaders and faculty should understand that truly inclusive workplaces are a byproduct of equitable practices that allow all members of the team to thrive regardless of whether they are in the minority or majority group. True inclusivity is modeled from the top down, and leaders should set these expectations for their employees.

Practice Cultural Humility

Cultural humility entails a lifelong commitment to self-evaluation, introspection, and reflective discernment of one's biases and privileges that may influence power imbalances with people from other groups (Tervalon & Murray-Garcia, 1998). Cultural humility is important because it provides the avenue for developing mutually beneficial partnerships that preserve and celebrate the cultural uniqueness of people from different groups (AACN, 2021). To effectively practice cultural humility, one must be dedicated to lifelong learning.

Pursue Allyship

Allyship is a relatively new concept, but one that I believe has been practiced for centuries to address the inequities experienced by minoritized groups. Nicole Asong Nfonoyim-Hara defines *allyship* as "when a person of privilege works in solidarity and partnership with a marginalized group of people to help take down the systems that challenge that group's basic rights, equal access, and ability to thrive in our society" (as cited in Dickenson, 2021, para. 2). For allyship to be effective, allies must be in positions of influence and should have power to effect change.

Nonetheless, anyone can be an ally. The most important traits of allies are unconditional support and advocacy for minoritized groups. Allies should also keep an open mind; they shouldn't assume that they know the answer to identified problems but should instead work collaboratively with the individuals they support to come up with solutions that are mutually acceptable.

While allyship is a great start, some scholars argue that we need to move beyond allyship to antiracism (Smith, 2021). I believe this is a pragmatic and necessary step to ensure that people do not simply end at allyship. Smith also suggests moving toward *emotional maturity*, which is the notion that we need to "'grow up and grow out' of racist ways of thinking, being, and doing." I agree that we have the capacity to do more, and we should admonish people to go the extra mile. In fact, the National Commission to Address Racism in Nursing report (2021) also provides a list of 10 ways to be antiracist in nursing. These include becoming story catchers, being genuine, managing ourselves, maximizing curiosity and minimizing certainty, distributing power, preserving the dignity of others, exposing unwritten rules, stopping labeling of others, supporting authenticity, and managing perceptions.

In my experience, for many people who are new to this movement, this may be a significant jump from their comfort zone. Perhaps by starting with becoming an ally, these experiences may provide the knowledge, skills, and resources to address racism later, directly through antiracism initiatives. Therefore, as the Chinese proverb says: A journey of a thousand miles begins with a single step. So, we should encourage people to take the first step, with the hope that they too will one day be antiracist.

> *"If you are neutral in situations of injustice, you have chosen the side of the oppressor."*
>
> –Desmond Tutu, winner of the 1984 Nobel Prize for Peace

Organizational-Level Strategies to Counter Othering in Academia

In addition to the strategies discussed previously, the National League for Nursing Diversity and Inclusion Toolkit (NLN, 2017) offers recommendations to counter othering and racism at the organizational level. These include requiring DEI training for organizational leadership as well as employees, developing and implementing a DEI strategic plan, incorporating diversity practices in the hiring process, and providing individualized resources and supports for minority faculty.

An organization should have a clear mission and vision that incorporate diversity and inclusivity as priority areas because the mission and vision will inform the DEI strategic planning and implementation.

I would like to draw our attention to incorporating diversity practices in our hiring processes. This will ultimately increase diversity in the workplace and serve as a springboard for all the other strategies and initiatives we have discussed.

Incorporating Diversity Practices in the Hiring Process

Historically, the intent of diversity hiring was to provide opportunities for individuals from marginalized and minoritized groups to have equal chances at advancement by reducing bias in the hiring process (Mondal, 2020). However, diversity hiring has been misconstrued to now mean that minorities and individuals from other marginalized groups are offered positions for which they do not qualify. This perception leads to animosity and treatment of affected individuals as inferior, which inadvertently leads to othering.

Education at all levels of the organizational structure is needed to understand that incorporating diversity practices in the hiring process does not spell out disenfranchisement of the dominant group. Rather, diversity practices level the playing field for all qualified candidates to receive equal consideration and access to opportunities and resources that are necessary for professional growth and development.

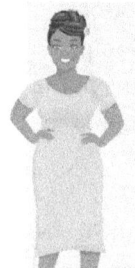

MERCY'S MOMENTS

I had just started my new position as a tenure-track assistant professor and was enjoying getting to know my new colleagues. One day, a colleague and I started talking about how difficult tenure-track positions are to come by these days. It was during this conversation that my colleague said to me, "Well, you probably didn't have to worry about getting a job since you are Black, and now all the universities are trying to increase their diversity numbers."

I was surprised by this comment because it implied that Black people and other minorities are not hired based on merit but because of a combination of factors that are independent of their qualification for the position—one of them being to increase the diversity profile of the organization. While some institutions do this, to simply assume that someone was hired only to meet a certain benchmark for the institution is both biased and demeaning.

Unfortunately, I'm not the only minority faculty who has ever been considered a "diversity hire" in its negative connotation by a colleague or two. This perception, if not corrected, has the potential to predispose the faculty member who is considered a diversity hire to maltreatment and passive-aggressive behaviors that are aimed at making them feel inferior.

AACN (2021) argues that when it comes to diversity, equity, and inclusion, simply having a policy is not enough. More needs to be done to ensure that the day-to-day practices and operations of the organization reflect attention to and prioritization of DEI initiatives. Relatedly, Rebecca Knight (2018) suggests seven practical ways to reduce bias in the hiring process:

- Seek to understand the hiring prejudices that are inherent in your organization's hiring processes.
- Rework your job descriptions by eliminating biased language and emphasizing collaborative and cooperative language.

- Go blind for the resume review to remove implicit bias in the process. Research has shown that people with mainstream names receive more callback for job opportunities compared to individuals with unique names (Bertrand & Mullainathan, 2003; Kline, Rose, & Walters, 2021).

- Give a work sample test as this is the best indicator for future success.

- Standardize the interview process to minimize bias and promote objective evaluation criteria based on attributes that directly impact work performance.

- Consider how likability is affecting the hiring process. Sometimes it is important to like the people you will be working with; however, likability should not supersede qualifications for the job an individual is applying for. At times, a faculty member of color may not be hired because some people just did not like them.

- Set diversity goals and measurable performance metrics to ensure that your organization is not simply putting policies in place, but actually practicing and incorporating these policies in everyday operations.

Individual-Level Strategies to Counter Othering in Academia

While we may not necessarily have the power or influence to personally change the systems and societal structures that perpetuate othering in academia, there are certain things we can do on an individual level that can counter the effects of othering. We address each of them in the paragraphs that follow. This is by no means an exhaustive list, but it is comprehensive enough to give you some tools to counter othering and thrive in academia.

Maintaining Personal Integrity and Dealing With Personal Insecurities

Dealing with othering in academia as a minority faculty can be difficult and often demoralizing. However, I encourage you to maintain your personal integrity as these situations arise. Two wrongs don't make a right. This is the motto I have lived by when it comes to issues of racism and othering, whether in nursing or in society in general. It takes personal integrity and courage not to fall into the trap of making assumptions about others. Additionally, I encourage people to learn to deal with personal insecurities related to race. Some of these insecurities stem from imposter syndrome, which has been shown to affect minorities at a higher rate compared to their white counterparts (Ahmed et al., 2020). We address imposter syndrome more in Chapter 10. Some coping styles that may help include:

Self-protective coping is a broad concept, but it basically points to a coping mechanism that prioritizes self-care (Spanierman et al., 2021). We delve more into why taking care of yourself is important in Chapter 10. I believe self-protective coping is important because it has the potential to grow psychological capital, which is associated with increased self-care, resilience, optimism, and hope. Domingue (2015) suggests that this type of coping can increase pride in belonging to certain groups and encourages focusing on the strengths of those groups.

Collective coping, as proposed by Lewis et al. (2013), requires developing connections and support systems with other minority faculty, friends, and family to foster microaffirmations (Solórzano et al., 2020). *Racial microaffirmations* are "subtle verbal and non-verbal strategies People of Color consciously engage (with other People of Color) that affirm each other's value, integrity, and shared humanity" (Solórzano et al., 2020, p. 185). Furthermore, this type of coping also significantly increases social capital of minority faculty.

Resistance coping focuses on directly addressing microaggressions by confronting perpetrators. Resistance coping requires challenging white normative behaviors (Lewis et al., 2013). My advice for people who choose to utilize this coping mechanism is to understand that they may encounter resistance but need to be resilient and persistent until they see the change they desire.

Engaging in Equity-Minded Learning

The University of Southern California Center for Urban Education (n.d.) defines *equity-mindedness* as a mode of thinking and perspective through which practitioners bring to the forefront patterns of inequities among student populations. This approach is instrumental in helping students identify their own biases. Implementing equity-minded learning in nursing may help to nurture the next generation of nurses who promote and embrace diversity, equity, and inclusivity in the nursing profession and beyond.

It is important for faculty to create a safe and nonjudgmental environment in which this type of learning can occur. Bennett et al. (2019) propose a four-step process with the acronym ARTS (affirmation, reflection, teachable moment, and summary) as a framework for having sensitive racial conversations with students.

Affirmation—affirm students and acknowledge their desire to have these conversations.

Reflection—promote introspection and encourage discussions to explore experiences.

Teachable moment—take advantage of moments to provide feedback and substantiate experiences with the literature.

Summary—always summarize what has been discussed.

Obtaining a Mentor From a Minority Background

Mentorship is important at every stage of career development. In this book, we have explored mentorship in detail in several chapters. But as a minority faculty member, having a mentor who is also from a minority group is important. This person does not necessarily have to be your primary mentor. They don't even have to be in your specific academic unit—if you have to seek them out from a different department, that is acceptable. Their purpose is to help you navigate the academic environment while providing unique perspectives on issues that are important to you as a minority faculty. I often say that just like you have a need for mentorship, other faculty and students have the same needs. Wherever possible, I encourage minority faculty to look at whom in their life they too can mentor and support.

Be a Power Connector

My last strategy is to encourage you to be a power connector in your own right. We talked about power connectors in Chapter 3, and it seems like a farfetched idea for someone just transitioning into their academic role. But you will be surprised to learn how many people look up to you, even as a new faculty in academia. Having a heart to open doors for others and connect them with resources and networks enriches your personal experiences—but more importantly, it slowly but surely tears down the systemic and structural barriers that have long sustained inequitable practices toward minoritized groups in academia.

> **SUCCESS NUGGET**
>
> Working to become an ally is a lifelong pursuit that requires ongoing education and self-reflection. You don't need to be perfect! A commitment to being honest with yourself and a willingness to challenge the status quo can make a big difference.

Final Thoughts

Change takes time, but I know that through intentional collective efforts, we can and should advocate for a profession that raises everyone together and leaves no one behind—a profession that allows its members to thrive and not merely survive. We should fight together to dismantle systems of oppression and discrimination that intentionally disqualify certain groups, particularly within the academic setting. We also have to be reminded that to achieve equity, equality alone may not suffice. In the words of Dr. Martin Luther King Jr.: "Injustice anywhere is a threat to justice everywhere. We are caught in an inescapable network of mutuality, tied in a single garment of destiny. Whatever affects one directly, affects all indirectly."

9

STRESS MANAGEMENT 101

Stress is a real thing and self-care matters. I'll say it again—stress is a real thing and self-care matters! As nurses, we are often caring and altruistic people who know how to give of ourselves unconditionally. However, sometimes that leaves our tanks empty because we give and give until we are exhausted. You have to take care of yourself to promote your own mental health and well-being. If you are not able to do this, your mental health will suffer, your family and friendships might be affected, your work performance may deteriorate, and you will not be able to give your best to your students either.

As I mentioned previously, the transition to an academic role can be a stressful journey. As you begin to settle into your role, it sometimes seems like instead of things getting better, they actually get worse because of the additional pressures that come up as you juggle multiple roles and responsibilities. But do not fret! There are many strategies you can employ to have some level of normalcy in your life. Let's start by discussing the potential sources of stress in academia that you need to be aware of; that way, you can be vigilant in ensuring that you are prioritizing self-care.

Sources of Stress in Academia

In a study that examined sources of university faculty stress, Meng and Wang (2018) found that all university faculty, regardless of rank, reported moderate to severe levels of stress. They also found that age, professional ranking, and length of teaching were significantly related to occupational stress. According to this study, the major contributors of stress were scientific research, professional development, and administrative affairs.

In a different study, Walter Gmelch (1993) identified additional sources of faculty stress after interviewing over 4,000 faculty members from more than 100 institutions in the United States. Sources of stress in this study included lack of rewards and recognition, time constraints, professional identity development, and student interactions. He also found that married professional women experienced more stress related to time constraints and professional identity development.

The evidence is clear, and study after study shows that faculty stress is a significant issue. Let's delve into how these different sources of stress can impact your life and examine some potential solutions to these problems.

Teaching Assignment Overload

In Chapter 1, I touched on the issue of teaching assignments and how to calculate your teaching load. I also mentioned that in nursing academia, our teaching loads tend to be heavier than those of our counterparts from other colleges at the same university. Junior nursing faculty members from other universities have also told me that their teaching loads seem heavier than their counterparts in other departments at their respective institutions. This can be a significant source of stress because it leaves many faculty members feeling like they cannot catch up with their teaching. Ultimately, this affects other aspects of their job, such as research and scholarly productivity as well as service engagement. These excessive assignments often lead to faculty working longer hours and even taking work home. In fact, Delello and colleagues (2014) found that faculty members worked an average of 54.35 hours per week, with almost a third of these hours from home.

While there is little you can personally do to remedy the excessive assignments, you can develop better time management skills and learn to be OK with prioritizing what needs your attention immediately and what can wait. My hope is that nursing administrators continue to explore ways in which teaching loads for nursing faculty can be reduced to levels that might be similar with other departments to lessen the impact of this factor on nursing faculty stress and burnout.

Unfortunately, most of us get caught up in the cycle of wanting to have everything perfect and doing it right now. As long as it is not an extremely important task that needs your immediate attention, it can wait. Another strategy to resolve this issue is to review your commitments. In Chapter 4, I mentioned that sometimes we get overcommitted with service, and that can easily derail you and take your time from other teaching responsibilities. Practice conscientious offloading, and you might find that there are a few extra hours in your day that you can reprioritize or even use for self-care needs.

Peer Competition

Academics tend to be labeled overachievers because they are always looking for the next big thing. I like to call us passionate because it's the spirit of inquiry and discovery that usually drives us to excel in our areas of expertise. However, this quest for excellence at all cost, every time, can sometimes lead to individuals competing with each other, especially for recognition. As highlighted by Gmelch (1993), lack of recognition and reward is a significant source of stress in academia.

Unhealthy peer competition can lead to sabotage and high levels of stress, especially among junior faculty members who may constantly feel the pressure to perform and produce. Now more than ever, this might be a difficult issue to deal with in academia because of the emphasis on data-informed metrics. For example, the college has metrics it has to meet related to enrollment and retention, passing rates, research and scholarship benchmarks, and so on. Oftentimes, the push to meet these metrics leads to peer competition because faculty members who are seen as contributing to these metrics are often publicly recognized.

The best antidote to this issue is knowing and accepting who you are. When you take the time to understand your purpose and goals, you will begin to focus on what *you* need to do to get where you aspire to be and not where everyone else is going. Unhealthy competition stems from trying to outdo someone whose mission and purpose are so different from yours. In fact, the danger in this approach is that you will miss working on your own priorities because you are concentrating on being better than someone else. You may have a completely different path in life. My daddy always told me that I am my own competition. I should strive to be a better version of who I was yesterday—not a better version of someone else.

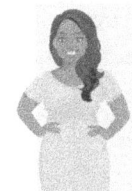

MERCY'S MOMENTS

When I first moved to the United States as an 18-year-old freshman in college, it was difficult learning about a new culture and trying to figure out who I was and what I wanted to be. One day, I was complaining to my daddy about the problems I was having with my transition. He said something that has stuck with me and has been a guiding principle not just in my personal life but also in my professional life. He said, "Mercy, God created you with all the passions, aspirations, and desires that are uniquely matched with all your skills, gifts, and talents that are required for you to achieve your purpose and mission in life. Every time you compete with or try to be someone else, you are creating a void in the universe that only you can fill—so why try to be someone else?"

Younger people or junior faculty are more prone to this source of stress because they are still discovering who they are and deciding what they want to be known for. I believe that sometimes as emerging scientists, we may feel that it may be easier to do research others are already doing than to take the time to figure out what we want out of our lives and chart our own course. One way you can prevent this from happening is what I suggested in Chapter 6—create a personal strategic plan and focus on growing personally and meeting your own goals and objectives, regardless of what everyone else is doing.

Unrealistic Personal Expectations

Unrealistic personal expectations sometimes come from perfectionism. I have often heard people say that many academics they know are Type A personalities. And honestly, this is not bad. You kind of need to be a Type A or have some traits of a Type A personality to thrive in an academic role. The problem is that sometimes this leads to overestimation of abilities, resources, and availability of time—hence, setting unrealistic personal goals.

Sometimes unrealistic personal goals can stem from feelings of being unworthy or not enough. These feelings lead people to set goals that are too high because they feel like that is the only way they can measure up. They measure their worth by their performance. We talk more about imposter syndrome in Chapter 10.

Unrealistic personal expectations can also be an extension of peer competition. People feel the need to outdo each other, and because of that, they tend to overextend themselves and set unrealistic goals. They become frustrated with themselves when they do not reach these goals, which can be a significant contributor to poor self-esteem because they are constantly failing at something.

So how do we solve this problem? A thorough examination of both internal and external factors that are contributing to your success is important in helping you set realistic goals. Additionally, looking at your life holistically will guide you in determining what is feasible, given your other professional and personal obligations.

Consistently setting unrealistic personal goals will lead to chronic stress and poor mental health outcomes. In my own research on nurses with substance use disorders, stress at work is a frequently cited reason for impaired practice and substance use problems (Mumba, 2018; Mumba, Baxley et al., 2019; Mumba, Kramer et al., 2019). That is why I'm so passionate about helping nurses acknowledge the stressors in their lives, find evidence-based approaches to coping with stress, and prevent substance misuse.

Power Dynamics Within the College

In Chapter 3, I introduced the concept of formal and informal hierarchies in academia. These hierarchies tend to create power dynamics among faculty holding different ranks within the college. Individuals holding the rank of assistant professor, especially those on tenure track, are the most affected by this source of stress (Gmelch, 1993; Meng & Wang, 2018). Often, the knowledge that someone else could potentially determine whether or not you progress in your career can be a significant source of stress. Unfortunately, these issues have been identified in academia for decades.

Although not much can presently be done to change the power dynamics in academia, my best advice to deal with this stress is to know the policies and procedures governing various aspects of your job, including evaluation, tenure, and promotion. Your college will have expected benchmarks for performance for each of the positions I discussed earlier in the book. Your job is to make sure you are meeting, at the very least, the minimum requirements for your position. It's wonderful if you can exceed expectations—just be mindful not to set unrealistic goals as that will bring a different source of stress in your life.

Additionally, make sure you are aware of mediation or arbitration processes both at the college level and the university level. Hopefully, you will not need to use these avenues, but if you feel there might be some discrimination involved in your work and you are not being fairly treated, then you are within your legal rights to pursue mediation or arbitration. I would personally like to say that these should be last resorts because if there is a culture of retaliation at your college or university, you must be absolutely certain that you have all the documentation to substantiate your claims before proceeding.

Student Interactions

Sometimes student interactions can be a source of stress, especially during the early days of transitioning to your academic role. You just want to do everything right, and you want your students to appreciate the work you are putting in to make sure they are getting a world-class education. Most students are very appreciative of their faculty members, but occasionally, you may run into a few students who stress you out. Yes, I said it. There are some students who will make you say a prayer or meditate before you go to the office. It's all part of the job.

What I see sometimes is that new faculty members fail to recognize or even do not want to admit that they have a difficult student. For some reason, they think this might reflect poorly on them. They suffer in silence until the pressure is too much to handle. I just want to say that you are not a bad teacher if you have a difficult student.

Also, I'm not sure if this is for the best or for the worst, but I have personally witnessed a trend in academia that when a conflict arises between a faculty member and a student, the student's version of the story is often given more weight than the faculty member's version. This is something a lot of my colleagues from around the country have mentioned to me. While it is important to be sensitive to student needs and complaints, I believe that faculty should be supported when the evidence shows that the student is in the wrong. Sometimes this lack of support from administrators and supervisors leads new faculty to suffer in silence for fear of being reprimanded.

This leads me to my next point. Sometimes faculty members tend to overextend themselves because they don't want students to poorly evaluate them at the end of the semester. In Chapter 2, I talked about Student Opinion of Instructor (SOI) scores. Unfortunately, sometimes students use these avenues to retaliate against faculty they do not like, whether for good reason or not. Therefore, faculty—and especially new faculty—may be reluctant to correct students for fear that they will receive poor student evaluations, which may negatively affect their job.

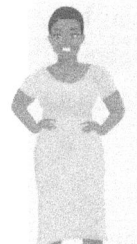

MERCY'S MOMENTS

I sometimes see new faculty bend over backward to appease their students because they don't want a bad evaluation. Over the few years that I have been teaching, I have come to realize that students appreciate a faculty member who holds them accountable and nurtures their abilities by stretching their capacity into realms they did not think possible. I remember comments like, "Dr. Mumba, you never let us get away with anything. We know that when you are teaching, we have to pay attention." My students sometimes call me tough, but they know I have their best interests at heart. I give them my time, I provide them with resources, and I always make sure they have the opportunity to be successful in my courses. But they still know that they have to do their work and come prepared for class, and they won't get a cheat sheet from me for the exam.

My student evaluations have been overwhelmingly positive. Yes, I occasionally get a comment about something one or two students did not like. But overall, my students think I'm a great teacher, even though they will admit that I'm tough—in a good way. The point I'm trying to put across is that although you want your students to succeed, accommodating unrealistic requests can easily make you spiral out of control and lose focus of the big picture. And honestly, not every student will like you, just like in real life.

When students are frustrated about something, evaluate the situation. If you conclude that you did everything possible to help them meet their learning objectives, let it go. If necessary, you might try escalating the grievance to the course leader (assuming it's not you) or your supervisor to help reach a resolution. But do not take every negative interaction with a student personally. If it was truly your fault, admit your shortcomings, learn from the situation, and move on.

Managing Stress Related to Interpersonal Dynamics

When you work with people from different backgrounds and diverse values, beliefs, and opinions, conflict is bound to arise. If you don't like the people you work with, it's quite hard to enjoy your work.

Sometimes people just don't get along—their personalities may be different, or it could even stem from issues such as peer competition, which I talked about earlier. Either way, it's important to understand conflict resolution principles and how to apply them.

In their research, Gillin Oore and colleagues (2015) suggest a two-pronged approach to conflict resolution in the workplace. They posit that there are individual factors and organizational factors that promote conflict resolution.

Conflict Resolution and the Individual

Several factors can influence conflict resolution on the individual level (Gillin Oore et al., 2015), including:

- Cognitive flexibility
- Emotional regulation
- Appropriate balance of self–other focus
- Fit of the person to the conflict situation

Cognitive Flexibility

Cognitive flexibility is the ability to adapt behaviors and thinking based on the environment. When you are adaptable, you are less likely to be overwhelmed when conflict arises because you can quickly adjust expectations, find solutions, and redirect energies. When you exercise cognitive flexibility, you don't have an insensate need to be right or to have the last word; therefore, you can agree to disagree and move on from a situation. I have to say, though, that agreeing to disagree is not always the best course. Learning to assert yourself in situations without being condescending to the other person is also very important.

> **SUCCESS NUGGET**
>
> When you exercise cognitive flexibility, you don't have an insensate need to be right. This strategy has the ability to disarm the person who is on the offensive. Most of the time, when both people in the conflict want to be right, the conflict drags on longer than it should. By taking the high road and agreeing to disagree, the other people will be left with the choice to either let it go or continue fighting. But if they continue fighting when the other person is not responding to their provocations, everyone will soon realize that they are the one instigating the conflict. This will help you maintain your integrity, and in the long run, people will see the other person as the problem.

Emotional Regulation

Emotional regulation is another tool you can utilize to resolve conflict. *Emotional regulation* refers to the ability to manage feelings. Sometimes when we encounter conflict, we lead with our emotions, based on how we are feeling in the moment. However, most of us know that if we take time to calm down, we will probably respond in a different way than if we reply at the height of the conflict. Having control over your emotions allows you to take time to reflect and introspect, determine how your actions may have contributed to the conflict, and brainstorm possible avenues for resolution.

Maybe this is not scientific at all, but exercising emotional regulation is important in creating boundaries with individuals who tend to be passive-aggressive and get their way by invoking negative emotions out of others—or as we like to say on the other side of town, don't let nobody push your buttons. There is a lot of literature that supports the utility of emotional regulation and its impact on setting health boundaries.

In her book, *Set Boundaries, Find Peace: A Guide to Reclaiming Yourself,* Nedra Glover Tawwab explores various aspects of setting boundaries. Topics include the cost of not having healthy boundaries, the six types of healthy boundaries, and strategies to identify and communicate your boundaries. I highly recommend this read as it will arm you with strategies for emotional regulation as a result of successfully implementing appropriate boundaries.

Self–Other Focus

Having a healthy balance of self–other focus is also important because it allows you to see the conflict from the other person's perspective. If we just take the time to see the conflict through the eyes of the other person, we may find that the seemingly insurmountable conflict can be easily resolved.

I also recommend not letting conflict fester without being addressed. The longer the conflict is allowed to continue, the more opportunities there are for associated issues to creep in and magnify minor conflict. This is a lesson I had to learn the hard way.

MERCY'S MOMENTS

About 10 years ago, a friend of mine and I had a disagreement about something minor. We both felt that we were right, and the other was wrong. Weeks and months went by without coming to a resolution. I noticed that as the months went by, more issues that were either tangentially related to the initial offense and others that were not even associated with the initial offense kept creeping into the conflict.

Before we knew it, a simple issue that we could have solved immediately led to a broken friendship that could have been salvaged if we both had taken the time to see the issue from the other person's perspective. Although we eventually reconciled, that relationship has never been the same. Since then, I learned that trying whenever possible to see the conflict through another person's eyes can help resolve conflict sooner and preserve the relationship.

This is especially important in the workplace because we spend so much time with our coworkers. We want to have a work environment in which we feel comfortable and get along with people. Conflict at work can be a significant stressor and, if not managed, can even lead to people leaving a job.

Fit of the Person to the Conflict Situation

The last aspect to consider is the fit of the person to the conflict solution. Sometimes people have different approaches to conflict resolution. In fact, research has shown that almost 50% of the variance in conflict resolution is attributed to the fit of the person to the conflict situation (Elfenbein et al., 2008). The types of conflict resolution styles include competing, collaborating, compromising, avoiding, and accommodating (Kilmann, 2021). Understanding your own style as well as the other person's style will help guide you as you approach the conflict resolution situation.

Below are some tips for having difficult conversations with colleagues (Bailey, 2021; Sousa et al., 2020):

- Keep an open mind.
- Self-reflect prior to difficult conversations.
- Keep the big picture in mind, and pursue collaboration.
- Show grace and understanding.
- Understand but don't suppress your own feelings about the situation.
- Focus on your own contribution to the conflict.
- Reframe the conflict resolution session into a learning conversation.

Conflict Resolution and the Organization

Gillin Oore and colleagues (2015) also suggest a second group of strategies that are at the organizational level. These include individual training on conflict resolution skills, workgroup conflict training, and formal mediation processes if the situation is warranted. In addition, I believe that organizations that promote a robust and authentic employee diversity, equity, inclusion, and belonging (DEIB) agenda provide an environment in which diversity of thought, beliefs, values, and opinions is appreciated. This promotes a culture of acceptance, thereby reducing the likelihood of "othering" people whose opinions are different from those of most faculty members. *Othering* means to "view or treat (a person or group of people) as intrinsically different from and alien to oneself" (The Oxford English Dictionary, n.d.-e). We explored this concept in greater detail and its harmful consequences for faculty who are "othered" in Chapter 8.

Work-Life Balance to Prevent Burnout

I recently found out that the World Health Organization (WHO) has officially included burnout in its International Classification of Diseases (ICD). The WHO defines *burnout* as:

> A syndrome conceptualized as resulting from chronic workplace stress that has not been successfully managed. It is characterized by three dimensions: 1) feelings of energy depletion or exhaustion; 2) increased mental distance from one's job, or feelings of negativism or cynicism related to one's job; and 3) reduced professional efficacy. Burn-out refers specifically to phenomena in the occupational context and should not be applied to describe experiences in other areas of life. (WHO, 2019, para. 4–6)

Burnout is not a new issue in academia, but little has been done to address this detrimental disorder (Fowler, 2015). Our culture sometimes glamorizes overworking and sees burnout as normal. With the COVID-19 pandemic, people have finally paid attention to the importance of mental health. We've finally been encouraged to stop wearing burnout as a badge of honor.

In her article "Why Do We Wear Exhaustion as a Badge of Honor?" Alicia Potts (2020) chronicles what has led to the unhealthy culture of being overworked and sleep-deprived. Some of the reasons cited include society glorifying busyness and associating it with success; the integration of technology into our everyday life, which makes work accessible to us 24/7; and equating sleeplessness with productivity. So how do we overcome this ingrained culture? I believe striving for work-life balance—or work-life integration, as some now call it—is the key.

Work-life balance has to be a personal priority as well as an organizational priority. Work-life balance will look different for everyone. Knowing what it means for you and your family is the most important thing. Alan Kohll (2018) suggests that employers focus on creating flexible work environments. The Canadian Center for Occupational Health and Safety (CCOHS, 2021) defines flexible work arrangements as "alternate arrangements or schedules from the traditional working day and week (para. 1)."

Flexible work environments for faculty may include the ability to work remotely when being in the office is not necessitated, availability of a compressed workweek, and extended leave days (e.g., maternal and paternal leave). This is especially true as younger generations join academia at higher rates. For example, millennials are more likely to leave a job that does not provide for work-life balance (Reiljen, 2016). If we cannot lessen the impact of burnout, we will always have to deal with attrition and severe faculty shortages, which simply exacerbate an already dire situation.

SUCCESS NUGGET

Work-life balance will look different for everyone. Knowing what it means for you and your family is the most important thing. Remember that your personal and family needs are just as important as your professional needs.

MERCY'S MOMENTS

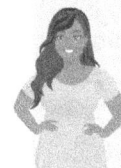

As I have grown as a researcher and scientist, I have come to appreciate the need to care for myself and prioritize my health and family time. I have learned that busyness does not always equal productivity. I have also realized that I tend to be a workaholic. Work comes naturally to me, and most of the time, it doesn't feel like work. I love and enjoy what I do, but that doesn't mean I should work seven days a week. As I took time to reflect and introspect, I realized that I come from a family with a very strong work ethic, and in my family, you always give 100%. In my second year on tenure track, my husband pointed out that I was consistently overworking. We all know that there are seasons when work is busy and you have to put in a little extra time and effort, but 24 hours a day, 365 days a year is unsustainable.

During that time, he bought me Michelle Obama's book, *Becoming*. He bought me this book because he knew I idolize Michelle. I just think she has such a wonderful story as a very successful minority woman in America. As I read the book, I realized that life is a balancing act. Many strong and ambitious women maintain brilliant professional careers without sacrificing their personal lives, but they must **choose** to have this balance.

I believe that most of us compartmentalize our lives, as if there are four versions of us—Mercy the professional, Mercy the wife, Mercy the daughter and sister, and Mercy the friend. Maybe you have even more categories than I have listed. But if Mercy the professional is doing great, and Mercy the daughter and sister is drowning, eventually one will have to give, and our lives will be incomplete.

As I read *Becoming*, I realized how often Michelle Obama practiced conscientious offloading—even though she did not call it that. I also noticed that I was more eager to practice conscientious offloading to accommodate other professional endeavors but not so much my personal and family endeavors. Now I'm more intentional with my rest, but it takes deliberate effort. Yes, I have to try not to work.

The more I've learned to rest, the more I'm actually basking in everything that I'm doing and becoming. It gives me the opportunity to be grateful for every single accomplishment and happening—and not simply glossing over to the next big thing. This is also an area of my life that one of my mentors was very intentional in helping me realize. With every interaction I have with her, she makes sure she asks me how I'm doing in my personal life. She is a staunch advocate for work-life balance, and she lives it out in her day-to-day life. She believes that I shouldn't just be an exceptional scientist, but I should be an exceptional human being. And I couldn't agree more with her.

Final Thoughts

One way you can achieve work-life balance is to rediscover what invigorates you, and make time for those activities (or people). For example, I love traveling to new places and learning about other cultures and how people live in different parts of the world. So, I made it a point to plan a couple of trips a year that were not work-related, where I could just take time off and wander the world.

Of course, COVID-19 made this more difficult in the past few months, but the point I'm trying to make is that you have to rediscover your passions outside your professional goals. When you first transition to an academic role, life may be stressful, and you may need to dedicate a little more time to your work than you normally would. But don't let that become a serial pattern.

My advice to you is to remind yourself that steady wins the race. Remember that setting unrealistic goals is one of the major contributors to stress at work. Take your time; you are running your own race and not in competition with anyone else. Stress is a real thing; it starts and ends with you. Therefore, take care of yourself—mind, body, and soul. You will thank me later.

10

THRIVING IN ACADEMIA

You have made it to the last chapter of the book, thriving in academia. My hope is that you have learned some strategies that you can use to help you successfully transition into your academic role. However, I don't want our journey together to end with transitioning into academia; I want you to thrive. This chapter is dedicated to exploring some concepts that may help you thrive in academia.

The word *thrive* means to flourish or prosper (Oxford English Dictionary, n.d.-f). There are certain concepts, such as resilience, grit, a growth mindset, and overcoming the imposter syndrome that may contribute to your ability to thrive in academia. Did you know that there is a whole branch of psychology called positive psychology? It is concerned with the study of the strengths and characteristics that enable individuals and communities alike to thrive (Positive Psychology Center, n.d.). We delve into each of them throughout the chapter. At the end of this chapter, I share with you some pearls of wisdom from people who have had successful careers in academia. I think you will appreciate their words of wisdom. So, let's dive in!

Resilience: The Glue That Holds Everything Together

I like to call resilience the glue that holds everything together because it represents a person's ability to bounce back from setbacks, which are quite common in academia and can often be demoralizing. Sometimes our lives feel like a million puzzle pieces. It is easy to get lost in the chaos of academia, even if it's organized chaos—and that is where resilience comes in. According to the American Psychological Association (APA), *resilience* is "the process of adapting well in the face of adversity, trauma, tragedy, threats, or significant sources of stress—such as family and relationship problems, serious health problems, or workplace and financial stressors" (APA, 2020, para. 4).

I find the APA's choice of words—adapting well—quite intriguing. Does this mean there is the potential to not adapt well? I did a little digging. APA defines *negative adaptation* as "a gradual loss of sensitivity or weakening of response due to prolonged stimulation" (APA, n.d., para. 1). You could adapt negatively to academia—accept its flaws as normal and learn to merely exist within the negative environment because you are tired of trying to make systemic changes. That is not what resilience is. With resilience, you push through the negative emotions and circumstances to find solutions to obstacles.

Building Resilience

We know that resilience is needed to adapt well to adversity, tragedy, threats, trauma, and significant sources of stress. The good news is that resilience is not a personality trait that only a select few individuals have. Rather, it involves particular thoughts, behaviors, and actions, which means that anyone can cultivate or build resilience. But how do we build resilience? APA (2021) suggests several approaches, including building connection, fostering wellness, finding purpose, embracing healthy thoughts, and seeking help.

In Chapter 3, we discussed the value of making connections and building your network. Human beings are relational—we often draw strengths from the relationships we build if they are personally meaningful. Taking the time to nurture the right relationships at work may increase your resilience because you will have people you can depend on in difficult times. People love going to work when they have meaningful friendships and relationships that go beyond the work environment. Additionally, through these meaningful relationships, you may grow your networks, which might unlock other resources you need to thrive in academia.

Having meaningful relationships, whether with your coworkers or other people in general, gives you a safety net of people who you can trust when you are going through difficult times and who can help when you are struggling to meet deadlines. Building these connections allows you to bounce back from challenging times when they come.

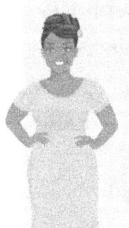

MERCY'S MOMENTS

About two years ago, I lost my brother to pancreatic cancer. He passed away in the middle of the academic semester. He had been in and out of the hospital for a few months prior to his passing, and I shared this with the ladies in the church small group I attended that semester. I had been in three other church small groups with these ladies and had built some really strong connections with them. I'm a spiritual person, and my faith is important to me. I remember our group praying that my brother would be healed and his health would be restored. When that did not happen and he passed, I was very crushed.

> On top of all that, it was the middle of the semester. At the time, I was serving as the course leader for the Fundamentals in Professional Nursing Course. This is one of the most time-consuming undergraduate courses in our college; it has a theory component and a clinical component. I was leading a team of 15 other faculty with 116 students in the course. A month prior to this, I had received the notice of award for our R61/R33 grant from NIH. As the principal investigator (PI), I was very busy setting up this award.
>
> My brother was still living in Zambia at the time of his passing, and I traveled for his funeral. I remember the brokenness I felt flying all the way there. It's almost a 22-hour flight (without counting connection time). Thankfully, my coworkers were so gracious. They offered to take over the lectures I was supposed to give and made sure the course continued to run smoothly while I was away for two weeks. When I came back to work, I found they had bought me a peace lily as a remembrance for my brother. The ladies in my church small group also checked on me regularly and prayed with me at each of our weekly meetings. The support I received from both my coworkers and the ladies in my church small group was the reason I was able to get through that difficult situation in my life. And, I have many stories that I can share about other difficult situations that I only got through because of the meaningful relationships I built with people around me.

Another strategy you can use to build resilience is fostering wellness. When you take care of your mind, body, and soul, as discussed in Chapter 9, you learn to adapt well to adversity and other challenges that come your way. Moreover, chronic stress impairs judgment. Research shows that when people are rested, they make better decisions and fewer mistakes and are more productive (Whitney et al., 2015; Whitney et al., 2019).

Other ways to foster wellness include maintaining a proper diet, staying hydrated, and exercising (Arida & Teixeira-Machado, 2021). Fostering wellness in your life will yield dividends in productivity and resilience, and here's why. When you make good decisions, you feel more confident about the potential outcomes, thereby relieving stress and ultimately increasing your resilience. On the contrary, when you consistently make bad choices, you make poor decisions that often result in failure. This is a concept that I'm embracing more as I grow older, and I hope you will too.

Finding your purpose and embracing healthy thoughts can also help build resilience. According to the Oxford English Dictionary (n.d.-g), *purpose* is "the reason for which something is done or created or for which something exists." So why do you exist? Have you ever asked yourself that question? Purpose is often mistaken for success in a certain field. However, you can be successful at something that you are not necessarily created to do. The reason why it is important to make this distinction is that success does not always bring fulfillment. Feeling fulfilled in what you are doing can help build resilience because even when you fail, you are more eager to try again if you believe that what you are doing is in line with your purpose in life.

Research has further shown that people who report high levels of eudemonic well-being, which is associated with a sense of purpose and self-actualization, live longer (Kobau et al., 2010). Additionally, people who have a sense of purpose make more money (Hill et al., 2016) and report fewer medical problems such as heart attacks and poor sleep (Musich et al., 2018). I believe that this is because a sense of purpose allows people to adapt well to whatever life throws at them, which increases their likelihood to bounce back and be resilient.

Similarly, having a sense of purpose can help you think positive thoughts. The French philosopher Rene Descartes said, "I think, therefore I am." Whatever you think and believe about yourself is what will happen. If you think positive thoughts, you are more likely to bounce back from setbacks because you do not think of an incident of failure as defining your entire existence. We touch more on this topic when we discuss the power of the growth mindset.

According to the U.S. Preventive Medicine (n.d.), some strategies to think more positive include:

- Paying attention to your own thoughts
- Nourishing your body and mind
- Giving back and helping others
- Building your inner confidence
- Creating affirming lists
- Talking back to your negative thoughts

A Growth Mindset

Embracing healthy thoughts is another source of resilience, according to the APA (2020). The way we think about ourselves impacts how we feel about ourselves and ultimately influences our perception of our ability to achieve goals and objectives. A few years ago, I participated in a leadership academy sponsored by the Southern Nursing Research Society (SNRS). As part of that program, we read the book *Mindset: The New Psychology of Success*, by Carol Dweck (2016). As I read some of the pages, I felt almost embarrassed—it was as if she was talking about me.

Many of us in academia have adopted a fixed mindset rather than a growth mindset. Dweck defines a *fixed mindset* as a belief that all our abilities are set in stone. The *growth mindset*, on the other hand, is the belief that you have the ability to adapt and acquire new skills; it's about being a perpetual learner (Dweck, 2016).

Adopting a growth mindset allows you to have room to fail, learn from experiences, and grow from the lessons that come as you stumble through life. You deal more effectively with change because challenges are viewed not as obstacles but as opportunities. With this mindset, you are better able to bounce back because you understand that no one situation defines your whole life. We are all a combination of successes, failures, challenges, and opportunities. How we perceive these issues determines whether we will give up or continue pushing until we reach our destination. So I encourage you to continue pushing if you believe you are living in your purpose.

Ask yourself how your fixed mindset may be hindering your ability to grow and flourish in your academic role. You may not have a fixed mindset in all areas of your life. Explore those areas in which you are not utilizing a growth mindset to maximize your successes. The secret to a growth mindset is that learning never ends, and perfection is never the destination. If you look closely, you will discover areas in your life that could use a sprinkle or two of the growth mindset—and that is how you build resilience.

Adopting a Strengths-Based Approach

Donald Clifton, who has been dubbed the father of strengths-based psychology, defines *strength* as the ability to consistently provide near-perfect performance (Clifton, 2007). In his view, strength is a product of talent (a natural way of feeling, thinking, and behaving) and investment (time spent practicing, developing your skills, and building your knowledge base; Clifton, 2007).

> CLIFTON'S STRENGTHS-BASED FORMULA
>
> Strength = Talent (a natural way of feeling, thinking, and behaving) x Investment (time spent practicing, developing your skills, and building your knowledge base).

Let's break this down.

Strengths require being proactive in gaining new knowledge in your desired area of interest, continuing to practice so you can improve your skills, and periodically evaluating your performance. Notice that the goal of utilizing a strengths-based approach is not to attain perfection but rather to increase the likelihood of achieving positive outcomes (Clifton, 2007).

A strengths-based approach involves three stages: identifying the strength, integrating the identified strengths into how individuals view themselves, and changing behavior to match the strength (Hodges & Clifton, 2004). This approach stems from understanding that we all have weaknesses and areas that need improvement. Rather than spending too much time trying to fix the weak areas, we should maximize outcomes by capitalizing on our strengths.

Taking a strengths-based approach has the potential to alleviate anxiety that arises when people fixate only on their weaknesses. It also gives you more flexibility in how you address your weaknesses because your performance or successes are not dependent on being a well-rounded, amazing person who can do everything. Releasing yourself from this pressure builds confidence, improves self-efficacy, and promotes general well-being, all of which contribute to building your resilience.

SUCCESS NUGGET

When I took the quiz, my top five strengths, in no particular order, were relator, strategic, learner, achiever, and responsibility. As I began learning more about these strengths, what they represent, and how I can utilize them to optimize my potential, I started to understand why I am the way I am. This allowed me to lead with my strengths in different situations and in different arenas. I call it understanding what makes me tick. This understanding enables you to harness positivity and buy-in from people whose support you need to move to the next level in your professional and personal life. Taking a strengths-based approach has been a game-changer for me. I recommend that you take this profile and create a plan on how you will use your strengths to take you to the next stage of your career.

Grit

Grit is another concept that is closely related to resilience. Angela Duckworth (2016), defines *grit* as a combination of passion and perseverance. Duckworth believes that talent alone is not enough to ensure success. You have to be passionate about what you do and persevere through the difficult times.

Have you met some really intelligent people who you felt were not living up to their potential? And have you met some so-called "average people" who have ended up being very successful? This can be equally true in academia. I often tell people not to be intimidated by people we consider smart. Remember the concept of a growth mindset? You may not be as naturally talented as the person next to you, but if you are passionate about what you do, you will soon discover that your passion, coupled with perseverance, will take you very far.

I first picked up Duckworth's book *Grit* as a new tenure-track assistant professor. I was trying to be proactive in ensuring that I had several tools in my toolbox to help me smoothly transition into my academic role. I had heard horror stories about academia, but I was determined to thrive regardless of the environment I was in. That conviction came because I was passionate about growing as a scientist and an educator. The concept that "effort counts twice" is one that has stuck with me. As you journey through your academic career, remember that your effort, coupled with all your skills and talents, will help you achieve your goals and thrive in academia. In fact, I often tell people that I'm not the smartest person you will ever meet, but I am one of the most dedicated people you will ever meet. And that, I believe, has been one of the secrets to my success so far. I suppose it has something to do with the dynamic combination of strengths I possess (achiever, responsibility, learner, strategic, and relator).

If you have not read this book, I highly recommend putting it on your to-read list. Reading this book made me realize that things take time to materialize. And here is something you should know too—your academic career is not a sprint; it's a marathon. Growing your grit will be essential to finding purpose in your work, fulfillment in everyday activities, and hope in the difficult times. And as the saying goes, "Showing up is half the battle."

Imposter Syndrome

To thrive in academia, you have to learn strategies to deal with imposter syndrome. *Imposter syndrome* entails an internal experience of intellectual inadequacy and unworthiness (Clance & Imes, 1978). In its simplest form, imposter syndrome is self-doubt that makes someone think that they are not good enough. This can be a common feeling during the transition phase into academia, and even the most confident people occasionally have this feeling. Imposter syndrome can lead to poor mental health such as depression, anxiety, stress, and lack of self-confidence (Clance & Imes, 1978).

Glover (2021) notes that imposter syndrome may be more apparent during transition periods. Additionally, imposter syndrome is more prevalent among individuals from minority and underrepresented groups (DiversityInc, 2019). Proactively developing strategies to respond to these feelings, whether constant or occasional, will help you thrive in academia. Sherman (2013) offers the following suggestions on how to deal with imposter syndrome:

- Pay attention to your feelings and evaluate whether they are empowering or disabling.
- Make a list of your strengths.
- Discuss your feelings with a trusted mentor.
- Accept that aiming for perfection is unrealistic and costly.
- Know that every new stage in your career requires you to develop new competencies.

- Be willing to be uncomfortable and work through the feelings.
- Focus on building competence.

The most important takeaway is that as you develop and grow into various levels of your career progression, these feelings are bound to come up. Consistently use the strategies listed above and remember that growth doesn't happen in the comfort zone. Working through your feelings with a trusted mentor or friend and persevering through the uncertainty will help you thrive.

Mentoring

Mentorship is the cornerstone of nursing advancement and is associated with higher levels of job satisfaction and retention (Horner, 2020). Having a mentor can teach you how to avoid pitfalls such as working in silos, procrastination, overextension of obligation, impostor syndrome, misinterpretation of data, and poor networking skills.

In nursing school, you are assigned a preceptor to shadow and give you feedback on your progress to help you improve. This should be consistent practice throughout our nursing professional careers. Navigating academia can be difficult and, frankly, frustrating when doing it all alone. This is why I advise establishing a mentor as soon as possible. Some institutions will assign you a mentor, while others will not. When you enter the uncharted waters of academia, having a tour guide or GPS is certainly an advantage. Earlier in the book, I shared with you how much I appreciated having first-year mentors when I started my current position.

Speaking of mentors, some of my long-term mentors wrote a book titled *Mentoring Today's Nurses: A Global Perspective for Success*. In this book, Susan Baxley, Kristina Ibitayo, and Mary Lou Bond (2014) list some qualities of good mentors, including:

- Supportive encouragement and honest feedback
- Availability of mentor for both formal and informal meetings
- Serving as guide for necessary behavior change
- Dependability
- Emotional intelligence
- Self-assuredness in mentor's own ability

I would also like to add to this list the importance of congruency in values and belief systems. Although it is still possible to be mentored by someone who does not share your values and beliefs, dissimilar views can become an insurmountable barrier and may lead to dissolution of the mentoring relationship.

As we discussed in Chapter 3, it is also vital to have at least one mentor who is a power connector. This is instrumental in helping you quickly build your network and gain credibility among other academics and scientists in your field. It further allows you to expand your professional network and collaborators at an exponential rate. It is important to note that as the mentee, you are equally responsible for the success of the mentoring relationship. According to Baxley et al. (2014), some of the ways in which you can support the mentoring relationship include being receptive to feedback and following through with any guidance provided by your mentor.

A caveat to this is that you will not always agree with your mentor. One thing, though, that I always did when I wanted to go a different route from what my mentors recommended was to let them know my rationale for taking that approach. Eventually, they saw my perspective and appreciated the respect I showed for them and their expertise by taking the time to explain why I thought another route was better for me and my trajectory. This is the power of open and honest conversation that comes only through building a genuine relationship with your mentors.

To establish a good mentor/mentee relationship, it is important to be receptive to constructive criticism and new opportunities. It is vital that you keep an open line of communication with your mentor to truly benefit from the relationship.

Here are a few tips to maintain the mentoring relationship once established:

- Establish a frequency for meeting regularly.
- Ask your mentor what time of day works best for them.
- Discuss your career goals.
- Discuss your strengths and weaknesses.
- Discuss how you have envisioned your trajectory of advancement.
- Understand your mentor's research area.
- Make a list of research topics that interest you.
- Stay up to date, follow their achievements, and congratulate your mentor.
- Follow up with your mentor on your advancement progress plan.
- Take notes so that you can educate and mentor someone else in the future.

Sometimes a mentoring relationship doesn't work. Perhaps they:

- Don't share your vision for success
- Don't want the responsibility of being a mentor

- Are new to mentoring and may be struggling to anticipate your needs
- Approach things differently from what works for you

If the relationship isn't working, it's time to have a conversation about what needs are not being met and why. This may simply be a rough patch, or the person may no longer be able to serve as your mentor. No matter the reason, it is still your responsibility to either reclassify this relationship (we talked about this in Chapter 3) or respectfully terminate the relationship.

Finding Your Own Mentor

Contrary to popular belief, it is not necessary to wait for mentorship to come to you. If you are seeking a mentor or have developed an interest in someone in your field, initiate that connection. Write that email. Request that LinkedIn connection. Request a lunch meeting. The worst thing that could happen is that they say no.

Additionally, you have to remember that it's OK to have multiple mentors for different aspects of your personal and professional life. The secret to having multiple mentors is clearly defining the purpose of the mentorship with each mentor. You are a complex human being, and no one individual is able to provide all the mentorship you need. In fact, it would be unfair to place that much responsibility on one person's shoulders.

BEING A MENTOR TO YOUR STUDENTS AND OTHERS WHO ARE JUNIOR TO YOUR ROLE

As you become more comfortable in your academic role, don't take too long before you take the opportunity to mentor your students and other faculty who are in more junior roles compared to yours. You have a lot of experience, gifts, and talents to share. The whole notion of giving back is so rewarding. Oftentimes, you will find fulfilment in helping someone else have a smoother transition into academia than you did.

A study by Miner (2019) that qualitatively explored the successful transition experiences of clinical nurses into their academic role found that one of the positive aspects of the transition related to giving back to the next generation. I have found that I also learn from the people I mentor, my students, and colleagues alike. My experiences are enriched by my interactions with my mentees, and for me, that is the successful model for mentoring.

MERCY'S MOMENTS

For this final Mercy's moment, I decided to take a different approach. As I wrap up this chapter and discussion about mentoring students and faculty in more junior roles, I invited one of my mentees to write about her mentoring experience for this book. She is a young, enthusiastic, and promising academic who has so much passion and zeal for what she does. She is a dual-certified advanced practice nurse (psychiatric mental health and family nurse practitioner).

Mentorship is such a powerful concept and has built my resilience as a person and professional. In the same way others have mentored me and opened doors for me, I am paying it forward in small but meaningful ways. Below, my mentee shares her story of the impact mentoring has had in her career so far.

When I began teaching fresh out of my doctoral program, I was under the impression that I had a comprehensive understanding of what teaching entailed. Little did I know that there were a lot of behind-the-scenes productions, collaboration, tasks, committees, and unspoken rules and expectations. It was like being in college all over again.

Others who were going through orientation with me seemed to be having a smooth transition and didn't have a ton of questions like I did. They seemed relaxed and calm. One day, a colleague mentioned that her mentor had made a helpful recommendation. A mentor, I asked? How do I get one? She told me that everyone gets a mentor when they are hired and told me where to look for mine.

Unfortunately, I had been overlooked and was not paired with a mentor. Almost two months into the first semester, I asked my supervising administrator to find a mentor for me, if possible. I likely would have eventually found my way through the tangled web of policy and procedures, meetings, manuscripts, and mania, but I'm sure I would have lost all of my hair in the process. That mentor made all the difference in my approach in just a few weeks of our connection.

The relationship continued to develop and made a huge impact on my assimilation to academia. She has advocated for me and given me advice on various aspects of my professional career. I am forever grateful for the knowledge and expertise she has shared with me and anticipate this will be a lifelong friendship. We still check in with each other regularly, collaborate on research, and congratulate each other on our newest accomplishments. In fact, I'm writing this book with her right now.

When looking for a new mentor, I recommend joining a local, state, national, and/or international chapter of a nursing organization (for example, Sigma Theta Tau International Honor Society of Nursing). Get to know people first, and develop a relationship with them before asking them to be your mentor. Joining a professional social media networking group, attending conferences, and following up with former instructors or faculty from your alma mater may be additional avenues to secure appropriate mentors.

Formal Resilience Training

Finally, I suggest that you receive formal training in resilience if you have not already done so. Research shows that people who have received training report better resilience compared to those who have not (Kunzler et al., 2020).

Final Thoughts

Life in general is full of challenges; I hope that you build the resilience to bounce back from the difficult times. You will have that stick-to-itiveness deep down in your belly because you understand your purpose and your mission. As Zig Ziglar says, "I don't care how much power, brilliance, or energy you have, if you don't harness it and focus it on a specific target and hold it there, you are never going to accomplish as much as your ability warrants." And while you're at it, make sure to celebrate every single win. After all, you are the only one who truly understands all the effort that went in to make it happen. Welcome to academia!

PEARLS OF WISDOM

Perceptions of flexibility matter. Academic jobs don't have regular hours. You are never or rarely finished with your work. Therefore, individuals need to establish appropriate work/life boundaries, such as when you will work evenings, weekends, or on vacation. This "freeness" of schedule enables you to have lunches with your children and participate in everyday tasks like going to the MD. Focus on the flexibility in creating your own schedule rather than "clocking out." Create your own routine.

"Publish or perish" manifests like any other anxiety. The anticipation is much worse than the actual process of gaining tenure. Relax. Breathe. Create a yearly plan as well as a five-year plan. Focus on small goals, and measure them by semester. Watch what you share with trainees as they spend a lot of time in grad school. Block time for thinking and writing into your schedule.

Gender and career stage matter when it comes to what is attractive or unattractive about an academic job. As a woman, create support networks that include other women in academia in positions of power.

Have mentors throughout all stages of your career. Welcome and reinforce learning from others, whether trainees, colleagues, or senior academics.

Pay it forward. Find and engage in what you *love* about academia, and then share that with others.

Rebecca Allen, PhD
Professor and Director, Alabama Research Institute on Aging
The University of Alabama

PEARLS OF WISDOM

Have a mentor or mentors from whom guidance can be sought and support can be obtained. It is helpful (maybe even critical) to have someone with whom questions and ideas can be processed. It can be easy, when transitioning into an academic role, to get derailed from focusing on advancing one's program of research. There are many activities, roles, and expectations that compete for a faculty member's time, creative energy, and focus. A mentor can help you to know when it is important to say "no" and when it is wise to say "yes." They can help you make decisions that will be in your best interest in the long term. Choose mentors wisely. Choose someone you can trust, and cultivate the relationship by connecting regularly so that through this trusting relationship, both mentor and mentee feel the freedom to question, challenge, and offer alternative solutions for consideration.

Work hard to maintain focus on advancing your program of research. Once in a faculty role, you no longer have your dissertation chair and others who prod you to move forward. While some of those relationships may remain, you will be more independent in your work, and the more you can be your own motivator, guide, and encourager, the better! Establish habits early on related to writing, goal setting, and monitoring your progress. Search for strategies that will help you maintain your focus.

Avoid saying "yes" to the many exciting offers and opportunities that come your way. Wisely choose a limited number of things you agree to do that are not a required part of your role. It can be easy to fill up your calendar/time with "shiny" opportunities that do not advance your program of research.

Carefully guard your time allocated to scholarship, and use it for advancing your scholarship!

Robin Bartlett, PhD, RN
Associate Dean for Research
Capstone College of Nursing
The University of Alabama

PEARLS OF WISDOM

When a nurse begins a new path in academia, it is important to search for a mentor, or more than one, to help guide you toward your goals to become a nursing scholar. Trust and freedom to discuss your path are essential in providing a give-and-take relationship as a way forward. You should also continue to develop a professional network to expand your influence in professional/scholarly associations.

Susan Baxley, PhD, MS, RN
Retired

PEARLS OF WISDOM

Navigating the many facets of academia can be daunting for a new faculty member and even more so for one on a tenure track, which some call the "crazy train." The first year on a tenure track can be overwhelming as a new faculty member tries to fully comprehend the responsibilities and expectations regarding teaching, research, and service. Therefore, it is important for a new faculty member to meet regularly with their immediate administrator (i.e., department chair, assistant dean) and any additional administrators (i.e., associate dean for research, dean, chair of Tenure and Promotion Committee) to clarify role expectations and to review written guidelines in the faculty handbook, annual assignment letters, college policies and procedures regarding evaluations, teaching support and research support, and tenure and promotion guidelines. A full comprehension of these will serve as a strong basis from which to proceed. Additionally, it is very important to the success of a tenure-track faculty member to establish and build a strong mentorship team. Some colleges or schools help to facilitate the establishment or assignment of at least one mentor for research or teaching. However, it is the responsibility of the faculty member to build their own mentorship team composed of one to two mentors who can provide guidance with the development of their research trajectory and who might possibly serve as members of the research team, if expertise aligns, and another mentor who can serve as a teaching mentor. It is also important for junior faculty to develop an individual development plan or scholarship trajectory plan. This document will serve as the scholar's blueprint for success and can be likened unto an individual strategic plan for one's career. This plan should include both short-term and five-year goals for teaching and research and include detailed plans and activities to achieve those goals, such as planned abstract, manuscript and grant submissions, and target deadlines. It can also include plans for professional service and leadership goals; however, it is important for junior faculty to not get bogged down or consumed with too much service. In academia, there are many more opportunities and requests for service participation than there are invitations to collaborate on manuscripts and grants. Therefore, two additional important skills for a junior faculty to hone are the ability to say, "no thank you" or "my schedule does not allow for that right now" and the ability to prioritize goals and responsibilities. It is also important to note, however, if a scholar is intending to conduct quality and equitable community-engaged research, then there will be times that their presence and service will be necessary to aid their community partners. This will help strengthen the relationship with the community partners and the target population and also ensure that the academic-community collaboration is bidirectional and mutually beneficial.

Safiya George, PhD, APRN-BC, FAANP
Dean and Professor
Christine E. Lynn College of Nursing
Florida Atlantic University

PEARLS OF WISDOM

The world of academia has its own culture, complete with its own language, traditions, social norms, and communication patterns. During the first year, assume the role of an ethnographic researcher. Observe, participate, and ask questions of trusted key informants. An attitude of cultural humility will facilitate a smoother transition into the life of academia.

Patricia Benner, author of *From Novice to Expert,* provides a theoretical lens through which to consider your transition into academia. In clinical practice, you may be a proficient clinician or even an expert; however, in academia, you are a beginner. Recognize that tasks that will become routine with practice will take longer at first. Pay attention to how your textbook knowledge of teaching translates into practice. Learn the differences between nurse-patient relationships and teacher-student relationships. Be patient with yourself. Becoming an expert in an academic world will take time and experience.

In contrast to the traditional view of academia as being inflexible and resistant to change, academia today is a vibrant, evolving enterprise of discovery and innovation. Stay attuned to new technology, changing student demographics, and an external environment that demands accountability for our outcomes. As a leader in academia, take calculated risks. Be willing to try new approaches to teaching, working with teams, and meeting the needs of your community.

When I was asked how I had managed to stay at the same university for 25 years, I reflected on my career. I realized wise administrators and mentors never allowed me to become bored. About every four to five years, a new opportunity emerged. One time, I accepted the responsibility for developing and teaching a controversial new course in a revised curriculum. Another time, I was asked to coauthor a research book. As I gained experience, I applied to be an associate dean leading a new PhD program and later was asked to become an interim dean. Saying no to any of these opportunities would have robbed me of relationships and growth that made me who I am as an academic administrator.

Jennifer Gray, PhD, RN, FAAN
Dean, College of Professional Studies
Oklahoma Christian University

PEARLS OF WISDOM

Life as an academic nurse leader is a gift; embrace the journey with meaningful connections and gratitude for the opportunity to help save lives, transform communities, and inspire hope for those you serve to reach their full potential and thrive.

Here is what I say to our Big Blue Nursing Nation students, and it works for new faculty and staff too. I use the CATS acronym: Communicate effectively, Ask for help, Take care of self, and Stay focused!

Janie Heath, PhD, APRN-BC, FNAP, FAANP, FAAN
Dean and Warwick Professor of Nursing
University of Kentucky College of Nursing

PEARLS OF WISDOM

Aligning your research, teaching, and service will further your efforts exponentially. Focus on one area of research, and make sure the service you do provides exposure to avenues of research and networking with colleagues with similar interests. Always have one member of your team who is more experienced than you, especially when you are first starting out. One day, you will be the senior member of the team and better able to provide guidance to those less experienced than you.

Charleen McNeil, PhD, MSN, RN
Professor and Associate Dean for Academic Affairs
Fran and Earl Ziegler College of Nursing
The University of Oklahoma Health Sciences Center

PEARLS OF WISDOM

I went from clinical supervisor to my first teaching position with an MSN: Remember to be kind to students, especially with their writing skills. Don't expect them to be perfect writers since many of them have not had a lot of practice in writing formally. Use a red pen only sparingly! You do not need to prove your superiority through discouraging students. (Note: I think I discouraged some RN-BSN students from continuing with their degree because I criticized everything they wrote. I think I wanted to prove I was a better writer. I regret that now.)

From new PhD to assistant professor on tenure track without a post-doc: Find a good mentor who wants you to succeed, and ask for guidance on 1) teaching load and how much time to spend on course preparation, 2) outside professional activities to pursue, 3) committees to be on at school and university levels, 4) manuscripts to write, and 5) whom on faculty to avoid. Listen to everything your mentor says, have frequent meetings, and follow your mentor's guidance!

Elizabeth Reifsnider, PhD, RN, FAANP, FAAN
Professor
College of Nursing and Health Innovation
Arizona State University

PEARLS OF WISDOM

I came from a different country with a different language and distinct overall culture. Initially, my words or behaviors were perceived as impolite in my work environment when I did not intend them to be. For example, my way of dressing was seen as casual when I felt that it was appropriate. My touching was perceived as invasive when I was trying to be friendly; my laughter occasionally emerged as improper because my sense of humor was distinctive. Now I am bicultural; I worked hard, and it took me some years to help others understand me and my culture, while I worked on understanding them and their culture. I can easily say that my career success is due to my resilience skills, such as flexibility, self-awareness, and innovation/creativity, and all the peer mentors and professional mentors who have guided me into the journey of becoming an Associate Dean for Diversity and Inclusion. Nowadays, I use my personal experience as a minority faculty who transitioned into academia from a completely different country and culture to help others who are doing the same. I am proud to say that now my most significant role is to advocate for the inclusion of underrepresented students, faculty, and staff in academia.

Jeanne-Marie Stacciarini, PhD, RN, FAAN
Associate Professor
Associate Dean for Diversity, Inclusion and Engagement
College of Nursing - University of Florida

PEARLS OF WISDOM

First, set your goals, be persistent and flexible, and treat rejections and failures as part of your learning and growth and view them positively. Second, surround yourself with people who can inspire and challenge you but also celebrate with you, find more than one mentor, and make sure the number of mentors is a manageable size for you. You need to be able to manage your mentoring team. Be grateful for all your mentors and colleagues who help you grow, and say thank you. Third, critically appraise all feedback you receive just as you are critically appraising the research evidence. I see so many novice researchers take advice and change topics frequently—and sometimes go from one side of the extreme to the other side. Be respectful of different perspectives, but you don't have to take every piece of feedback you receive. After you critically appraise all the feedback, act on what you think fits you and your situation, and follow through. Explain and be ready to justify your choices. Even if you fail, don't regret your decisions; learn from them. Don't stop moving forward just because you have challenges or fail. Find a way to keep going, regardless. Fourth, stay focused. If you dive deeper into one topic and stick with it, you will achieve success more quickly. Lastly, academia is not an ivory tower, so connect research with real-world people, communities, and healthcare.

Jing Wang, PhD, MPH, RN, FAAN
Dean and Professor
Florida State University

PEARLS OF WISDOM

My advice to a new faculty member is find your niche in an area that fuels your passion, seek the advice of trusted mentors, and hold firm to your values.

Lovoria Williams, PhD, APRN-BC, FAANP, FAAN
Associate Director & Endowed Research Professor for Cancer Health Equity
Markey Cancer Center
Associate Director, UK Center for Clinical and Translational Science
Codirector, Integrated Special Populations
University of Kentucky, College of Nursing

PEARLS OF WISDOM

As a nurse academic, a great world awaits you! I have been able to find my passion and live it out as a nurse academic. I have always felt a great sense of excitement, curiosity, and commitment in this work and hope that you will too. I have found great reward, year after year, knowing I was engaged in meaningful work that promotes the good in our world. I have enjoyed sharing my passion for teaching and learning and psychiatric mental health nursing with students over the years. I hope that you too will find this enjoyment. I've been fortunate to work with all levels of professional nursing students, including baccalaureate, master's, and doctoral, as well as students from other disciplines (social work, psychology, higher education administration, human development, medicine, pharmacy). My research has provided me with data about the human condition. I am an advocate for science to guide practice. I see it as critical to advancing human and environment health and healing. So, my advice and pearls of wisdom are to find your passion, as I have done. My research and practice have given me opportunities to grapple with some of the complex health problems that members of our society face, especially in the aftermath of dehumanization, trauma, abuse, and violence, and research is one of my greatest passions. As an administrator, I get the wonderful opportunity to support not only students but also staff and faculty—and make connections with the larger body of alumni. Whether it is teaching, researching, practicing nursing, serving others, or forging new community engagements, I am in my element. I hope that you too will have this experience as a nurse academic!

Danny Willis, DNS, RN, PMHCNS-BC, CNE, FAAN
Joan Hrubetz Dean and Professor
Trudy Busch Valentine School of Nursing
St. Louis University

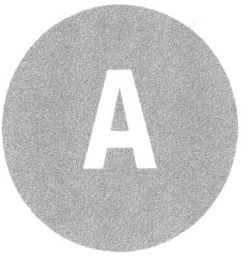

APPLICATION PROCESS

The application process for your entry-level academic position will vary based on the position you are interested in. Below is a sample application and interview process for a tenure-track assistant professor position. This process may vary from institution to institution but overall will be very similar.

You may be invited to apply for a position, or you may find a position by yourself and apply. Universities usually have a recruitment budget for faculty. The size of the budget may dictate what the college is willing to do to get you on board.

Before You Apply

1. Update your curriculum vitae.

2. Update your philosophy of teaching statement.

3. Update your research and scholarship trajectory statement.

4. Update your diversity, equity, and inclusion personal statement (this is increasingly becoming a requirement for many institutions).

Begin the Application Process

Most universities will require a formal application to be completed through their jobs site. Once your application is submitted, it is sorted by an HR specialist to ensure that you meet the minimum requirements for the position.

Once You Meet the HR Minimum Requirements

Your application will be forwarded to the college with all supporting documents. Most colleges have what is called a search committee. The search committee's responsibility is to ensure that you are a suitable candidate for the college, and they will work with college administration to determine whether to extend an interview.

The Interview Process

Once the college determines that they are interested in hosting you for an interview, you will correspond with someone from the search committee to determine a suitable date and time for the interview. If many individuals have applied for a limited number of positions, there may be a screening phase, whereby you interview with members of the search committee before they offer you an interview with the general faculty and staff.

If You Are Still Deemed a Suitable Candidate

You might be invited to the next phase of the interview process. This can be done in person or virtually. You will be provided with an itinerary of individuals to interview with at different times of the day, and this usually includes a research presentation for the faculty and administrators. This can last anywhere from 30 minutes to an hour, depending on the institution. Below are examples of individuals you may be required to interview with as part of the process:

1. The dean of the college of nursing

2. The senior associate dean of the college of nursing

3. The associate dean of research

4. The dean of undergraduate or graduate education (depending on where they think you will primarily teach)

5. Faculty and staff (you are usually required to give a presentation of 30 minutes to an hour about you and your teaching, research, and service backgrounds)

6. Student representatives

7. Other researchers on campus with whom you may potentially collaborate if you accept a position

If Your Interview Is in Person

You will be assigned a member of the search committee to host you for the duration of your interview process. Usually, in-person interviews also involve meeting several other people over lunch and dinner. The university will likely cover all travel costs if applicable (e.g., flights, accommodation, and meals).

As you can see, this can be a grueling day. Sometimes the interview process may last for two days. Be mentally ready and prepared for an exhausting process.

Once the Interview Is Complete

Most universities will allow faculty to provide feedback on whether they think you would be a good fit and a valuable member of the college if hired. The administrators often take this feedback into consideration when deciding whether to offer you the position. The ultimate decision, though, lies with the dean of the college of nursing.

If Your Interview Was Successful

The dean will reach out to you with an offer letter. You can negotiate the terms of the appointment if you are considering the position, or you can accept what is offered if you believe it is fair. Once the terms have been agreed upon and finalized, you can officially accept the offer of employment.

After You Accept the Offer

You will now work with HR to complete background checks. Usually, the offer is contingent on passing your criminal background checks and any other requirements by your institution.

Once all of this is done, congratulations and welcome to academia!

B

SAMPLE LESSON PLAN

Date: 01/15/2022
Topic: Acid-Base Balance
Class Time: 9am – 12pm

Class Objectives:
1. Describe the process involved in acid-base balance.
2. Examine common disturbances in acid-base balances.
3. Evaluate factors that affect normal acid-base balance.
4. Discuss clinical assessments of patients with acid-base imbalances.
5. Discuss clinical interventions appropriate for patients with various acid-base imbalances and their proper implementation.
6. Identify and evaluate nursing interventions for patients with acid-base imbalances.

Time	Activity	Materials
9:00am – 9:50pm	Lecture • Normal ABGs • Acid-base buffering system • Acid-base regulation • Respiratory acidosis • Respiratory alkalosis	PowerPoint Presentation
9:50am – 10:00am	BREAK	
10:00am – 10:20am	Interactive Class Quiz • At least one question per major concept covered • 10 total questions • Short Q&A with students to clarify any misunderstandings	Kahoot Quiz Platform
10:20am – 10:50am	Lecture (continued) • Metabolic acidosis • Metabolic alkalosis • Anion gap	PowerPoint Presentation
10:50am – 11:00am	BREAK	
11:00am – 11:20am	Interactive Class Activity • Work through at least one unfolding case study per concept covered in last section • Three case studies • Short Q&A with students to clarify any misunderstandings	Unfolding Case Studies

Time	Activity	Materials

11:20am – 11:40am	Lecture (continued)
	• Mixed disorders
	• Compensated states
	   a. Partially compensated
	   b. Fully compensated
		PowerPoint Presentation

11:40am – 12pm	Practice Questions • At least one question per major concept covered • 15 total questions • Short Q&A with students to clarify any misunderstandings	Kahoot Quiz Platform

Go to the Sigma Repository to download this as a reusable document. Follow the link or use the QR code to navigate to the Repository page.

http://hdl.handle.net/10755/22478

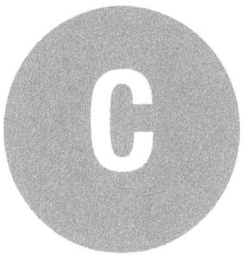

SERVICE COMMITMENT CONTACT HOURS

Go to the Sigma Repository to download this as a reusable document. Follow the link or use the QR code to navigate to the Repository page.

http://hdl.handle.net/10755/22478

Service Opportunity	Approximate Number of Hours per Month
College Service	
University Service	
Professional Service	
Community Service	
Total	

*Add more rows as necessary

REFERENCES

Abelson, J. S., Wong, N. Z., Symer, M., Eckenrode, G., Watkins, A., & Yeo, H. L. (2018). Racial and ethnic disparities in promotion and retention of academic surgeons. *American Journal of Surgery, 216*(4), 678–682. https://doi.org/10.1016/j.amjsurg.2018.07.020

Academia. (2013, February 26). *Is a "big ego" necessary for a tenure-track faculty position?* [Online forum post]. Stack Exchange. https://academia.stackexchange.com/questions/8221/is-a-big-ego-necessary-for-a-tenure-track-faculty-position

Ahmed, A., Kaushal, A. Cruz, T., Kobuse, Y., & Wang, Kristen. (2020, December 8). *Why is there a higher rate of impostor syndrome among BIPOC?* https://doi.org/10.5281/zenodo.4310477

Ajil, A., & Blount-Hill, K. L. (2020). "Writing the other as other": Exploring the othered lens in academia using collaborative autoethnography. *Decolonization of Criminology and Justice, 2*(1), 83–108. https://doi.org/10.24135/dcj.v2i1.19

American Association of Colleges of Nursing. (2020a, September). *Nursing shortage.* https://www.aacnnursing.org/news-information/fact-sheets/nursing-shortage

American Association of Colleges of Nursing. (2020b, October). *DNP fact sheet*. https://www.aacnnursing.org/News-Information/Fact-Sheets/DNP-Fact-Sheet

American Association of Colleges of Nursing. (2021). *Diversity, equity, and inclusion faculty tool kit 2021*. https://www.aacnnursing.org/Education-Resources/Tool-Kits

American Association of University Professors. (n.d.). *1940 statement of principles on academic freedom and tenure*. https://www.aaup.org/report/1940-statement-principles-academic-freedom-and-tenure

American Association of University Professors. (2006). *AAUP contingent faculty index*. https://www.aaup.org/sites/default/files/files/AAUPContingentFacultyIndex2006.pdf

American Association of University Women. (n.d.). *Fast facts: Women working in academia*. https://www.aauw.org/resources/article/fast-facts-academia/

American Council on Education. (n.d.). *An agenda for excellence: Creating flexibility in tenure-track faculty careers*. https://president.umd.edu/sites/default/files/2020-06/Tenure%20Flexibility%20Summary%2C%202005.pdf

American Psychological Association. (n.d.). Negative adaptation. In *APA dictionary of psychology*. Retrieved October 1, 2021, from https://dictionary.apa.org/negative-adaptation

American Psychological Association. (2020, February 1). *Building your resilience*. https://www.apa.org/topics/resilience

Anderson, N. (2021, June 16). Black professors push a major university to diversify and confront racism. *The Washington Post*. https://www.washingtonpost.com/education/2021/06/16/penn-state-Black-faculty-racism/

Arida, R. M., & Teixeira-Machado, L. (2021, January 20). The contribution of physical exercise to brain resilience. *Frontiers in Behavioral Neuroscience, 14*, 626769. https://doi.org/10.3389/fnbeh.2020.626769

Bailey, S. (2021, April 9). Seven steps for having difficult conversations. *American Nurse*. https://www.myamericannurse.com/seven-steps-for-having-difficult-conversations/

Baxley, S. M., Ibitayo, K. S., & Bond, M. L. (2014). *Mentoring today's nurses: A global perspective for success*. Sigma Theta Tau International.

Benner, P. (2001). *From novice to expert: Excellence and power in clinical nursing practice*. Prentice Hall.

Bennett, C., Hamilton, E. K., & Rochani, H. (2019). Exploring race in nursing: Teaching nursing students about racial inequality using the historical lens. *OJIN: The Online Journal of Issues in Nursing, 24*(2). https://ojin.nursingworld.org/MainMenuCategories/ANAMarketplace/ANAPeriodicals/OJIN/TableofContents/Vol-24-2019/No2-May-2019/Articles-Previous-Topics/Exploring-Race-in-Nursing.html

Bertrand, M., & Mullainathan, S. (2003, July). *Are Emily and Greg more employable than Lakisha and Jamal? A field experiment on labor market discrimination*. National Bureau of Economic Research. https://www.nber.org/papers/w9873

Bichsel, J., & McChesney, J. (2017, February). *The gender pay gap and the representation of women in higher education administrative positions: The century so far.* Research report. CUPA-HR. https://www.cupahr.org/wp-content/uploads/cupahr_research_brief_1.pdf

Blanchard, K. (2014, Januray 3). Are you dependable? *Chief Learning Officer.* https://www.chieflearningofficer.com/2014/01/03/are-you-dependable/

Boyer, E. L. (1990). *Scholarship reconsidered: Priorities of the professoriate.* The Carnegie Foundation for the Advancement of Teaching. https://www.umces.edu/sites/default/files/al/pdfs/BoyerScholarshipReconsidered.pdf

Brinkert, R. (2010). A literature review of conflict communication causes, costs, benefits and interventions in nursing. *Journal of Nursing Management, 18*(2), 145–156. https://doi.org/10.1111/j.1365-2834.2010.01061.x

Bucklin, B. A., Valley, M., Welch, C., Tran, Z. V., & Lowenstein, S. R. (2014, February 10). Predictors of early faculty attrition at one academic medical center. *BMC Medical Education, 14,* 27. https://doi.org/10.1186/1472-6920-14-27

Burton-Hughes, L. (2017, December 18). What is unconscious bias in recruitment? *Hub.* https://www.highspeedtraining.co.uk/hub/types-of-unconscious-bias/

Canadian Center for Occupational Health and Safety. (2021). *Flexible work arrangements.* https://www.ccohs.ca/oshanswers/psychosocial/flexible.html

Carnegie Classification of Institutions of Higher Education. (n.d.). *Basic classification description.* https://carnegieclassifications.iu.edu/classification_descriptions/basic.php

Carr, A. R. (2014). *Stress levels in tenure-track and recently tenured faculty members in selected institutions of higher education in northeast Tennessee.* Electronic Theses and Dissertations. Paper 2329. https://dc.etsu.edu/etd/2329

Center for Creative Leadership. (2022). *Inclusive leadership: Steps your organization should take to get it right.* https://www.ccl.org/articles/leading-effectively-articles/when-inclusive-leadership-goes-wrong-and-how-to-get-it-right/

Clance, P. S., & Imes, S. A. (1978). *The impostor phenomenon in high achieving women: Dynamics and therapeutic intervention.* http://mpowir.org/wp-content/uploads/2010/02/Download-IP-in-High-Achieving-Women.pdf

Clifton, D. (2007). *StrengthsFunder 2.0: Discover your CliftonStrengths.* Gallup. https://store.gallup.com/p/en-us/10385/strengthsfinder-2.0-(hardcover)

Cornell University. (2022). *Teaching philosophy statement.* https://gradschool.cornell.edu/career-and-professional-development/pathways-to-success/prepare-for-your-career/take-action/teaching-philosophy-statement/#:~:text=What%20is%20a%20teaching%20philosophy,why%20you%20teach%20that%20way

Cortisman, L. (2008). Experiences of African American students in a predominantly White, two-year nursing program. *Association of Black Nursing Faculty Journal, 19*(1), 8–13.

Cox, T. N. (2019). *Self-care isn't selfish: A busy woman's journey to self-care.* Emerald Design Co.

Crayton, D. (2019). Faculty of color at predominantly white colleges and universities. *Culminating Projects in Education Administration and Leadership, 63.* https://repository.stcloudstate.edu/edad_etds/63

Curle, C. (n.d.). *Us vs. them: The process of othering.* https://humanrights.ca/story/us-vs-them-the-process-of-othering

Daouk-Öyry, L., Anouze, A. L., Otaki, F., Dumit, N. Y., & Osman, I. (2014). The JOINT model of nurse absenteeism and turnover: A systematic review. *International Journal of Nursing Studies, 51*(1), 93–110. https://doi.org/10.1016/j.ijnurstu.2013.06.018

Delello, J. A., McWhorter, R. R., Marmion, S. L., Camp, K. M., Everling, K. M., Neel, J., & Marzilli, C. (2014). The life of a professor: Stress and coping. *Polymath: An Interdisciplinary Arts and Sciences Journal, 4*(1), 39–58. https://ojcs.siue.edu/ojs/index.php/polymath/article/view/2932

Detweiler, G. (2018, March 27). 10 expert social media tips to help your small business succeed. *Forbes.* https://www.forbes.com/sites/allbusiness/2018/03/27/10-expert-social-media-tips-to-help-your-small-business-succeed/?sh=15f3aac414a1

Dickenson, S. (2021, January 28). *What is allyship?* NIH Blog. https://www.edi.nih.gov/blog/communities/what-allyship

DiversityInc. (2019). *Imposter syndrome can take a heavy toll on people of color, particularly African American.* https://www.diversityinc.com/imposter-syndrome-can-take-a-heavy-toll-on-people-of-color-particularly-african-americans/

Domingue, A. D. (2015). "Our leaders are just we ourself": Black women college student leaders' experiences with oppression and sources of nourishment on a predominantly white college campus. *Equity & Excellence in Education, 48*(3), 454–472. https://doi.org/10.1080/10665684.2015.1056713

Duckworth, A. (2016). *Grit: The power of passion and perseverance.* Scribner.

Dweck, C. S. (2016). *Mindset: The new psychology of success.* Ballantine Books.

Edgoose, J., Quiogue, M., & Sidhar, K. (2019). How to identify, understand, and unlearn implicit bias in patient care. *Family Practice Management, 26*(4), 29–33. https://www.aafp.org/fpm/2019/0700/p29.html#fpm20190700p29-ut1

Edwards, N., & Roelofs, S. (2019). *Developing a program of research: An essential process for a successful research career.* CHNET Press.

Elfenbein, H. A., Curhan, J. R., Eisenkraft, N., Shirako, A., & Baccaro, L. (2008). Are some negotiators better than others? Individual differences in bargaining outcomes. *Journal of Research in Personality, 42,* 1463–1475. http://dx.doi.org/10.1016/j.jrp.2008.06.010

Fahkry, T. (2018, January 21). *Life is not happening to you, but responding to you.* Mission.org. https://medium.com/the-mission/life-is-not-happening-to-you-but-responding-to-you-7aad9f308e1c

Fang, D., Moy, E., Colburn, L., & Hurley, J. (2000). Racial and ethnic disparities in faculty promotion in academic medicine. *JAMA, 284*(9), 1085–1092. https://doi:10.1001/jama.284.9.1085

Flaherty, C. (2020, September 14). Burning out. *Inside Higher Ed.* https://www.insidehighered.com/news/2020/09/14/faculty-members-struggle-burnout

Folger, J. (2021). *The causes and costs of absenteeism.* https://www.investopedia.com/articles/personal-finance/070513/causes-and-costs-absenteeism.asp

Fowler, S. (2015). Burnout and depression in academia: A look at the discourse of the university. *European Journal for the Philosophy of Communication, 6*(2), 155–167. https://doi.org/10.1386/ejpc.6.2.155_1

Fyfe, M., Horsburgh, J., Blitz, J., Chiavaroli, N., Kumar, S., & Cleland, J. (2022). The do's, don'ts and don't knows of redressing differential attainment related to race/ethnicity in medical schools. *Perspectives on Medical Education, 11*(1), 1–14. https://doi.org/10.1007/s40037-021-00696-3

Gale, P. (2013). *Your network is your net worth: Unlock the hidden power of connections for wealth, success, and happiness in the digital age.* Atria Publishing Group.

Gillin Oore, D., Leiter, M. P., & LeBlanc, D. E. (2015). Individual and organizational factors promoting successful responses to workplace conflict. *Canadian Psychology/Psychologie canadienne, 56*(3), 301–310. https://doi.org/10.1037/cap0000032

Glanville, I., & Houde, S. (2004). The scholarship of teaching: Implications for nursing faculty. *Journal of Professional Nursing, 20*(1), 7–14. https://doi.org/10.1016/j.profnurs.2003.12.002

Glover, E. J. (2021). *Understanding imposter syndrome among nurses.* https://ajnoffthecharts.com/understanding-imposter-syndrome-among-nurses/

Gmelch, W. H. (1993). *Coping with faculty stress.* SAGE Publishing.

Gray, T. (2020). *Publish and flourish: Become a prolific scholar* (15th ed.). Starline Printing.

Greenwald, A. G., McGhee, D. E., & Schwartz, J. L. K. (1998). Measuring individual differences in implicit cognition: The implicit association test. *Journal of Personality and Social Psychology, 74*(6), 1464–1480. https://doi.org/10.1037/0022-3514.74.6.1464

Haider, A. H., Schneider, E. B., Sriram, N., Scott, V. K., Swoboda, S. M., Zogg, C. K., Dhiman, N., Haut, E. R., Efron, D. T., Pronovost, P. J., Freischlag, J. A., Lipsett, P. A., Cornwell, E. E., MacKenzie, E. J., & Cooper, L. A. (2015). Unconscious race and class biases among registered nurses: Vignette-based study using implicit association testing. *Journal of the American College of Surgeons, 220*(6), 1077–1086.e3. https://doi.org/10.1016/j.jamcollsurg.2015.01.065

Hall, J. M., & Fields, B. (2012). Race and microaggression in nursing knowledge development. *Advances in Nursing Science, 35*(1), 25–38. https://doi.org/10.1097/ANS.0b013e3182433b70

Hamric, A. B., Hanson, C. M., Tracy, M. F., & O'Grady, E. T. (2013). *Advanced practice nursing e-book: An integrative approach.* Elsevier.

Harrison, C., & Tanner, K. D. (2018). Language matters: Considering microaggressions in science. *CBE—Life Sciences Education, 17*(1), 1–8. https://doi.org/10.1187/cbe.18-01-0011

Hassouneh, D. (2006). Anti-racist pedagogy: Challenges faced by faculty of color in predominantly white schools of nursing. *Journal of Nursing Education, 45*(7), 255–262. https://doi.org/10.3928/01484834-20060701-04

Hassouneh, D., Lutz, K. F., Beckett, A. K., Junkins, E. P., & Horton, L. L. (2014). The experiences of underrepresented minority faculty in schools of medicine. *Medical Education Online, 19*(1), 24768. https://doi.org/10.3402/meo.v19.24768

Hill, P. L., Turiano, N. A., Mroczek, D. K., & Burrow, A. L. (2016). The value of a purposeful life: Sense of purpose predicts greater income and net worth. *Journal of Research in Personality, 65*, 38–42. https://doi:10.1016/j.jrp.2016.07.003

Hodges, T. D., & Clifton, D. O. (2004). Strengths-based development in practice. In P. A. Linley & S. Joseph (Eds.), *Positive psychology in practic* (pp. 256–268). John Wiley & Sons.

Horner, D. K. (2020). Mentoring: Positively influencing job satisfaction and retention of new hire nurse practitioners. *Plastic Surgical Nursing. 40*(3), 150–165. https://doi.org/10.1097/PSN.0000000000000333

Iheduru-Anderson, K., Okoro, F. O., Moore, S. S. (2022). Diversity and inclusion or tokens? A qualitative study of black women academic nurse leaders in the United States. *Global Qualitative Nursing Research.* https://doi.org/10.1177/23333936211073116

Jakes, T. D. (2016, May 24). *Confidants, constituents, and comrades* [Video]. YouTube. https://www.youtube.com/watch?v=2Y6N7wuG6JI

Jane. (n.d.). *Frequently asked questions.* The Biosemantics Group. https://jane.biosemantics.org/faq.php#how

Joseph, Y. D., & Davis, N. (2021). Implicit bias and caring in student nurses. *Journal of the National Black Nurses Association, 32*(2), 42–47.

June, A. W. (2015, November 8). The invisible labor of minority professors. *The Chronicle of Higher Education.* https://www.chronicle.com/article/the-invisible-labor-of-minority-professors/

Kilmann, R. (2021). *Thoman-Kilmann instrument.* https://kilmanndiagnostics.com/about/

Kline, P. M., Rose, E. K., & Walters, C. R. (2021, July). *Systemic discrimination among large U.S. employers.* National Bureau of Economic Research. https://eml.berkeley.edu//~crwalters/papers/randres.pdf

Knight, R. (2018). *7 practical ways to reduce bias in your hiring process.* https://www.shrm.org/resourcesandtools/hr-topics/talent-acquisition/pages/7-practical-ways-to-reduce-bias-in-your-hiring-process.aspx

Kobau, R., Sniezek, J., Zack, M. M., Lucas, R. E., & Burns, A. (2010). Well-being assessment: An evaluation of well-being scales for public health and population estimates of well-being among US adults. *Applied Psychology, 2*(3), 272–297. https://doi.org/10.1111/j.1758-0854.2010.01035.x

Kohll, A. (2018, March 27). The evolving definition of work-life balance. *Forbes.* https://www.forbes.com/sites/alankohll/2018/03/27/the-evolving-definition-of-work-life-balance/?sh=722adccc9ed3

Kraicer, J. (1997, May 5). *The art of grantsmanship.* https://www.hfsp.org/sites/default/files/webfm/Communications/The%20Art%20of%20Grantsmanship.pdf

Kunzler, A. M., Helmreich, I., Chmitorz, A., König, J., Binder, H., Wessa, M., & Lieb, K. (2020). Psychological interventions to foster resilience in healthcare professionals. *The Cochrane Database of Systematic Reviews, 7*(7), CD012527. https://doi.org/10.1002/14651858.CD012527.pub2

Lashuel, H. A. (2020). *Mental health in academia: What about faculty?* https://elifesciences.org/articles/54551

Lewis, J. A., Mendenhall, R., Harwood, S. A., & Huntt, M. B. (2013). Coping with gendered racial microaggressions among Black women college students. *Journal of African American Studies, 17*(1), 51–73. https://doi.org/10.1007/s12111-012-9219-0

Lexico. (n.d.). Conscientious. In *Lexico.com dictionary.* Retrieved February 2, 2022, from https://www.lexico.com/en/definition/conscientious

Loftin, C., Newman, S. D., Dumas, B. P., Gilden, G., & Bond, M. L. (2012). Perceived barriers to success for minority nursing students: An integrative review. *International Scholarly Research Notices,* 806543. https://doi.org/10.5402/2012/806543

Macmillan Dictionary. (n.d.). Othering. In *Macmillian.com dictionary.* Retrieved February 2, 2022, from https://www.macmillandictionary.com/us/dictionary/american/othering

Maslow, A. (1943). A theory of human motivation. *Psychological Review, 50*(4), 370–396. https://doi.org/10.1037/h0054346

Maslow, A. H. (1970). *Motivation and personality* (2nd ed.). Harper & Row.

McIntosh, P. (1989). *White privilege: Unpacking the invisible knapsack.* https://psychology.umbc.edu/files/2016/10/White-Privilege_McIntosh-1989.pdf

McKinsey & Company. (2021). *Women in the workplace – 2021.* https://wiw-report.s3.amazonaws.com/Women_in_the_Workplace_2021.pdf

Meng, Q., & Wang, G. (2018). A research on sources of university faculty occupational stress: A Chinese case study. *Psychology Research and Behavior Management, 11,* 597–605. https://doi.org/10.2147/PRBM.S187295

Menon, A. C., & Priyadarshini, R. G. (2018). A study on the effect of workplace negativity factors on employee engagement mediated by emotional exhaustion. The 3rd International Conference on Materials and Manufacturing Engineering. Kancheepuram, India. https://iopscience.iop.org/article/10.1088/1757-899X/390/1/012027/pdf

Merriam-Webster. (n.d.-a). Bias. In *Merriam-Webster.com dictionary.* Retrieved February 3, 2022, from https://www.merriam-webster.com/dictionary/bias

Merriam-Webster. (n.d.-b). Individuation. *In Merriam-Webster.com dictionary.* Retrieved February 3, 2022, from https://www.merriam-webster.com/dictionary/individuation

Miami University. (n.d.). *Defining, documenting, and evaluating service: A guide for regional campus faculty.* https://www.miamioh.edu/academic-affairs/admin-affairs/regional-faculty-service-guide/index.html

Miner, L. A. (2019). Transition to nursing academia: A positive experience. *The Journal of Continuing Education in Nursing, 50*(8), 349–354. https://doi.org/10.3928/00220124-20190717-05

Mondal, S. (2020). *Diversity hiring: 6 steps to hiring more diverse candidates.* Ideal blog. https://ideal.com/diversity-hiring/

Mumba, M. N. (2018). Employment implications of nurses going through peer assistance programs for substance use disorders. *Archives of Psychiatric Nursing, 32*(4), 561–567. https://www.doi.org/10.1016/j.apnu.2018.03.001

Mumba, M. N., Baxley, S. M., Snow, D. E., & Cipher, D. J. (2019). A retrospective descriptive study of nurses with substance use disorders in Texas. *Journal of Addictions Nursing, 30*(2), 78–86. https://www.doi.org/10.1097/JAN.0000000000000273

Mumba, M. N., & Kraemer, K. (2019). Substance use disorders among nurses in medical-surgical, long-term care, and outpatient services. *MEDSURG Nursing, 28*(2), 87–92. http://www.medsurgnursing.net/cgi-bin/WebObjects/MSNJournal.woa

Musich, S., Wang, S. S., Kraemer, S., Hawkins, K., & Wicker, E. (2018). Purpose in life and positive health outcomes among older adults. *Population Health Management, 21*(2), 139–147. https://doi.org/10.1089/pop.2017.0063

National Commission to Address Racism in Nursing. (2021). Summary Report: Listening sessions on racism in nursing. https://www.nursingworld.org/~49be5d/globalassets/practiceandpolicy/workforce/commission-to-address-racism/final-racism-in-nursing-listening-session-report-june-2021.pdf

National League for Nursing. (2017). *NLN diversity and inclusion toolkit.* https://www.nln.org/docs/default-source/uploadedfiles/default-document-library/diversity-toolkit.pdf

National Organizational of Nurse Practitioner Faculties. (2012). *Nurse practitioner core competencies.* https://www.aacn.org/~/media/aacn-website/certification/advanced-practice/npcorecompetenciesfinal2012.pdf?la=en

O'Neal, C., Meizlish, D., & Kaplan, M. (2019). *Writing a statement of teaching philosophy for the academic job search.* University of Michigan Center for Research on Learning and Teaching. https://crlt.umich.edu/sites/default/files/resource_files/CRLT_no23_revised.pdf

Oxford English Dictionary. (n.d.-a). *Invest.* Retrieved October 1, 2021, from https://www.oed.com/

Oxford English Dictionary. (n.d.-b). *Networking.* Retrieved October 1, 2021, from https://www.oed.com/

Oxford English Dictionary. (n.d.-c). *Opportunity cost.* Retrieved January 1, 2022, from https://www.oed.com/

Oxford English Dictionary. (n.d.-d). *White privilege.* Retrieved January 1, 2022, from https://www.oed.com/

Oxford English Dictionary. (n.d.-e). *Othering.* Retrieved January 1, 2022, from https://www.oed.com/

Oxford English Dictionary. (n.d.-f). *Thrive.* Retrieved January 1, 2022, from https://www.oed.com/

Oxford English Dictionary. (n.d.-g). *Purpose*. Retrieved January 1, 2022, from https://www.oed.com/

Parr, C. (2014, April 6). *Race discrimination in universities still a problem, reports survey*. https://www.timeshighereducation.com/news/race-discrimination-in-universities-still-a-problem-reports-survey/2012474.article?page=0

Peterson, N. B., Friedman, R. H., Ash, A. S., Franco, S., & Carr, P. L. (2004). Faculty self-reported experience with racial and ethnic discrimination in academic medicine. *Journal of General Internal Medicine, 19*(3), 259–265. https://doi.org/10.1111/j.1525-1497.2004.20409.x

Pfeifer, H. L. (2016). *How to be a good academic citizen: The role and importance of service in academia*. Taylor & Francis. https://www.tandfonline.com/doi/full/10.1080/10511253.2015.1128706?src=recsys

Phiri, A. (2018). Critical spaces: Processes of othering in British institutions of higher education. *Journal of Feminist Scholarship, 7*(7), 13–27. https://digitalcommons.uri.edu/jfs/vol7/iss7/4

The Physics Classroom. (n.d.). *Newton's Third Law*. https://www.physicsclassroom.com/class/newtlaws/Lesson-4/Newton-s-Third-Law

Pierce, C., Carew, J., Pierce-Gonzalez, D., & Willis, D. (1978). An experiment in racism: TV commercials. In Pierce C. (Ed.), *Television and education* (pp. 62–88). Sage.

Pololi, L., Cooper, L. A., & Carr, P. (2010). Race, disadvantage and faculty experiences in academic medicine. *Journal of General Internal Medicine, 25*, 1363–1369. https://doi.org/10.1007/s11606-010-1478-7

Pololi, L. H., Evans, A. T., Gibbs, B. K., Krupat, E., Brennan, R. T., & Civian, J. T. (2013). The experience of minority faculty who are underrepresented in medicine, at 26 representative U.S. medical schools. *Academic Medicine: Journal of the Association of American Medical Colleges, 88*(9), 1308–1314. https://doi.org/10.1097/ACM.0b013e31829eefff

Positive Psychology Center. (n.d.). *Our mission*. https://ppc.sas.upenn.edu/our-mission

Potts, A. (2020, March 13). *Why do we wear exhaustion as a badge of honor? On the glamorization of sleep deprivation in modern society*. Thrive Global. https://thriveglobal.com/stories/why-do-we-wear-exhaustion-as-a-badge-of-honour/

RegisteredNursing.org. (2021, July 26). *Nurse educator*. https://www.registerednursing.org/nurse-educator/

Renjen, P. (2016). *What makes young professionals walk out of their jobs?* https://www.weforum.org/agenda/2016/01/young-leave-jobs/

Robinett, J. (2014). *How to be a power connector: The 5+50+100 rule for turning your business network into profits*. McGraw-Hill.

Robinson, O. V. (2013). Telling the story of role conflict among Black nurses and Black nursing students: A literature review. *Journal of Nursing Education, 52*(9), 517–524. https://doi.org/10.3928/01484834-20130819-04

Rockquemore, K. A., & Laszloffy, T. (2008). *The Black academic's guide to winning tenure—without losing your soul*. Lynn Reinner Publishers.

Saad, L. (2022, January 12). *Military brass, judges among professions at new image lows*. Gallup. https://news.gallup.com/poll/388649/military-brass-judges-among-professions-new-image-lows.aspx

Sherman, R. O. (2013). *Imposter syndrome: When you feel like you're faking it*. https://www.researchgate.net/profile/Rose-Sherman/publication/256475007_Sherman_RO_2013_Imposter_Syndrome_American_Nurse_Today_85_57-58/links/0c960522f53cd9647f000000/Sherman-RO-2013-Imposter-Syndrome-American-Nurse-Today-85-57-58.pdf

Smith, R. (2021). Moving from allyship to antiracism. *Creative Nursing, 17*(1), 51–54. https://doi.org/10.1891/CRNR-D-20-00080

Solórzano, D., Pérez Huber, L., & Huber-Verjan, L. (2020). Theorizing racial microaffirmations as a response to racial microaggressions: Counterstories across three generations of Critical Race Scholars. *Seattle Journal for Social Justice, 18*(2), 185–216.

Sousa, B., Harder, L., & Clark, A. (2020). *Making difficult conversations easier: How to raise and resolve difficult academic work issues*. https://www.universityaffairs.ca/career-advice/career-advice-article/making-difficult-conversations-easier/

Spanierman, L. B., Clark, D. A., & Kim, Y. (2021). Reviewing racial microaggressions research: Documenting targets' experiences, harmful sequelae, and resistance strategies. *Perspectives on Psychological Science, 16*(5), 1037–1059. https://doi.org/10.1177/17456916211019944

Sreenivasan, S. (2017). *How to use social media in your career*. https://www.nytimes.com/guides/business/social-media-for-career-and-business

Stacciarini, J. R. (2002). Experiencing cultural differences: Reflections on cultural diversity. *Journal of Professional Nursing, 18*(6), 346–349. https://doi.org/10.1053/jpnu.2002.130166

Sue, D. W. (2010). *Microaggressions in everyday life: Race, gender, and sexual orientation*. Wiley.

Sue, D. W., Capodilupo, C. M., Torino, G. C., Bucceri, J. M., Holder, A. M., Nadal, K. L., & Esquilin, M. (2007). Racial microaggressions in everyday life: Implications for clinical practice. *The American Psychologist, 62*(4), 271–286. https://doi.org/10.1037/0003-066X.62.4.271

Sue, D. W., Lin, A. I., Torino, G. C., Capodilupo, C. M., & Rivera, D. P. (2009). Racial microaggressions and difficult dialogues on race in the classroom. *Cultural Diversity and Ethnic Minority Psychology, 15*(2), 183–190. https://doi.org/10.1037/a0014191

Sue, D. W., & Spanierman, L. B. (2020). *Microaggressions in everyday life* (2nd ed.). Wiley.

Sutcliffe K. M. (2011). High reliability organizations (HROs). *Best Practice & Research. Clinical Anaesthesiology, 25*(2), 133–144. https://doi.org/10.1016/j.bpa.2011.03.001

Tawwab, N. G. (2021). *Set boundaries, find peace: A guide to reclaiming yourself*. TarcherPerigee.

Teoli, D., Sanvictores, T., & An, J. (2021, September 8). *SWOT Analysis*. StatPearls. https://www.ncbi.nlm.nih.gov/books/NBK537302/

Tervalon, M., & Murray-García, J. (1998). Cultural humility versus cultural competence: A critical distinction in defining physician training outcomes in multicultural education. *Journal of Health Care for the Poor and Underserved, 9*(2), 117–125. https://doi.org/10.1353/hpu.2010.0233

Tochluck, S. (2010). *Witnessing whiteness*. Rowman & Littlefield Inc.

Tracy, M. F., & O'Grady, E. T. (Eds.). (2017). *Hamric and Hanson's advanced practice nursing: An integrative approach* (6th ed.). Elsevier.

Truong, K. A. (2021). *Why and how colleges should acknowledge the invisible labor of faculty of color*. https://www.insidehighered.com/users/kimberly-truong

Tuckman, B. W., & Jensen, M. A. C. (1977, December 1). Stages of small-group development revisited. *Group & Organization Management, 2*(4), 419–427. https://doi.org/10.1177/105960117700200404

University of Minnesota Center for Education and Innovation. (2021). *Writing your teaching philosophy*. https://cei.umn.edu/writing-your-teaching-philosophy

University of Southern California Center for Urban Education. (n.d.). *What is equity-mindedness?* https://cue.usc.edu/equity/equity-mindedness/

University of York. (n.d). *Academic citizenship*. https://www.york.ac.uk/admin/hr/pay-and-grading/promotion/citizenship/#:~:text=Academic%20citizenship%20covers%20activities%20additional,collegial%20operation%20of%20the%20institution

U.S. Preventive Medicine. (n.d.). *Positive psychology: Practicing the power of positive thinking*. https://www.uspm.com/tag/positive-thinking/

Western University Centre for Teaching and Learning (n.d.). *Writing a teaching philosophy statement*. https://teaching.uwo.ca/awardsdossiers/teachingphilosophy.html

Whitney, P., Hinson, J. M., Jackson, M. L., & Van Dongen, H. P. A. (2015). Feedback blunting: Total sleep deprivation impairs decision making that requires updating based on feedback. *Sleep, 38*(5), 745–754. https://doi.org/10.5665/sleep.4668

Whitney, P., Hinson, J. M., & Nusbaum, A. T. (2019). A dynamic attentional control framework for understanding sleep deprivation effects on cognition. *Progress in Brain Research, 246*, 111–126. https://doi.org/10.1016/bs.pbr.2019.03.015

Wilson, D. W. (2007). From their own voices: The lived experience of African American registered nurses. *Journal of Transcultural Nursing, 18*(2), 142–149. https://doi.org/10.1177/1043659606298611

World Health Organization. (2019, May 28). *Burn-out an "occupational phenomenon": International Classification of Diseases*. https://www.who.int/news/item/28-05-2019-burn-out-an-occupational-phenomenon-international-classification-of-diseases

Worthen, M. (2021, September 20). The fight over tenure is not really about tenure. *The New York Times*. https://www.nytimes.com/2021/09/20/opinion/tenure-college-university.html

Zamudio-Suarez, F. (2021, January 26). Race on campus: The mental burden of minority professors. *The Chronicle of Higher Education.* https://www.chronicle.com/newsletter/race-on-campus/2021-01-26?cid2=gen_login_refresh&cid=gen_sign_in

Zhou, M., & Brown, D. (2015). *Educational learning theories* (2nd ed). https://oer.galileo.usg.edu/cgi/viewcontent.cgi?article=1000&context=education-textbooks

Zsurzsan, A. (2014, February 20). *10 powerful quotes from industry leaders that will inspire you to empower your employees.* https://transcosmos.co.uk/blog/10-quotes-employee-empowerment/

INDEX

NOTE: Page references with an *f* are figures; page references with a *t* are tables.

A

AACN (American Association of Colleges of Nursing), 31, 149, 190
AANA (American Association of Nurse Anesthesiology), 154
AAUP (American Association of University Professors), 96, 97
abstracts, 131. *See also* publication(s); writing
academia
  adjunct positions, 10, 146
  administrative positions, 9–10
  application processes, 251–254
  appointments (*see* appointments)
  clinical-track assistant professors, 8–9
  collaboration, 49–50 (*see also* collaboration)
  Distribution of Effort (DOE), 19–22 (*see also* Distribution of Effort [DOE])
  high reliability organizations (HROs), 150–151
  instructor positions, 9
  length of appointments, 13–18
  managing roles, 15
  othering in, 169–170, 172–175 (*see also* othering)

pillars of, 5–6
power dynamics in, 210–211
reasons for leaving, 35
sources of stress in, 206–213 (*see also* stress management)
tenure-track assistant professors, 7–8
transitions to, 142 (*see also* clinical faculty roles)
types of entry-level appointments, 6–7
academic citizenship, 74–75, 164
  benefits of, 91
  definition of, 74–75
  joining professional organizations, 83, 84–85
  opportunities for, 74
  risk of overcommitment, 79, 86–90
academic roles, 4. *See also* educators
academic teaching, 27–29
  calculating workloads, 31*t*
  confidence-building strategies, 36–43
  evaluating effectiveness, 43–46
  managing workloads, 29–33
  practicality of teaching assignments, 33–34
  teaching assignment overload, 35–36
access to mentors, 105–107
adapting prior instructor's work, 41
adjunct positions, 10, 146
administration, 5–6
administrative positions, 9–10
advanced practice registered nurses (APRNs), 34, 151, 153, 160

adversity, adapting to, 224
affinity bias, 178
agencies, external funding, 105
alliances, choosing, 63–64
allyship, pursuing, 195–196, 202
American Association of Colleges of Nursing (AACN), 31, 149, 190
American Association of Nurse Anesthesiology (AANA), 154
American Association of University Professors (AAUP), 96, 97
American Council on Education, 98
American Psychological Association (APA), 224, 225
analysis, 55–57, 101. *See also* SWOT
anchoring bias, 179
antiracism, 195. *See also* racism
anxiety, 230
apartheid, 172. *See also* othering
application processes, 251–254
appointments, 6–7
  9-month, 14–18
  12-month, 13–14
  adjunct positions, 10, 146
  administrative positions, 9–10
  clinical-track assistant professors, 8–9
  commitments, 87 (*see also* commitments)
  Distribution of Effort (DOE), 19–22 (*see also* Distribution of Effort [DOE])
  instructor positions, 9
  length of, 13–18
  selecting positions, 10–13

special considerations of, 18–19
tenure-track assistant professors, 7–8
types of (*see* entry-level positions)
APRNs (advanced practice registered nurses), 34, 151, 153, 160
art, academic teaching as, 27–29. *See also* academic teaching
ARTS (affirmation, reflection, teachable moment, and summary), 201
assignments
  guest lecturing, 41–42
  practicality of teaching, 33–34
  teaching assignment overload, 35–36
assimilation, 194
Association of American Colleges and Universities, 96
assumptions, 171
attitudes, managing, 126

B

bachelor of science in nursing (BSN), 77
balance, work-life, 218–221
Baxley, Susan, 233
Becoming (Obama), 220
behaviorism, 38
benchmarks for promotions, 162
bias, 178–182
  awareness of, 179
  language use and, 198
  strategies to combat implicit, 180–182
  types of, 178, 179
The Black Academic's Guide to Winning Tenure—Without Losing Your Soul (Rockquemore/Laszloffy), 112
Black faculty, othering and, 173, 174, 175, 177, 178. *See also* faculty; othering
Blanchard, Ken, 58
Bond, Mary Lou, 233
Boyer, Ernest, 129
burnout, 32
  definition of, 218
  preventing, 218–221
  teaching assignment overload, 35–36

C

Canadian Center for Occupational Health and Safety (CCOHS), 219
candidates, suitable, 249
careers
  appointments (*see* appointments)
  clinical faculty roles, 141–149 (*see also* clinical faculty roles)
  managing roles, 15
  selecting positions, 10–13
Carnegie Classification of Institutions of Higher Education, 99
Center for Creative Leadership, 194

Center for Research and Scholarship, 106
certification requirements, 152, 158, 160
certified registered nurse anesthetists (CRNAs), 154, 155
certified registered nurse practitioners (CRNPs), 152
Circassia, ethnic cleansing of, 172. *See also* othering
citizenship. *See* academic citizenship
classifications of networking, 68–71
classrooms, confidence-building strategies, 36–43
Clifton, Donald, 229
clinical faculty roles, 141–142
   applying for promotions, 164–166
   calculating dollar value of time, 146–148
   choosing collaborative relationships, 151–157
   collaborative agreements, 151–157
   core competencies, 157–159
   distance to work, 148–149
   incomes, 144
   maintaining clinical expertise, 145
   organizational environments and, 149–151
   overview of, 142–149
   part-time *vs.* full-time, 145–146
   research, 161–164
   scholarship, 161–164
   specialty considerations, 159–161
   workloads and, 142, 144, 147
clinical-track assistant professors, 8–9, 142. *See also* clinical faculty roles
cognitive flexibility, 214–215
cognitivism, 38
collaboration, 49–50. *See also* networking
   building, 123
   choosing collaborative relationships, 151–157
   history of tenure track, 96–98
   negotiations, 154, 155–157
   relationships and, 153–154
   strategic classifications of, 68–71
   strategies, 57–64
collaborative agreements, 151–157
   negotiations, 154
   relationships (*see* relationships)
collective coping, 200
colleges. *See also* education; educators
   access to mentors, 105–107
   courses (*see* courses)
   culture, 103–104
   faculty member research, 103
   institutional research expectations, 99–101
   intramural seed funding, 104–105
   selecting college of nursing, 99–109
   service at the college-level, 75–77
   struggling with teaching and research, 110–111
   support, 101–103
   support from dean of research, 107–109

commitments
  conscientious offloading, 87–88
  contact hours, 89t–90t
  Distribution of Effort (DOE), 88–90 (*see also* Distribution of Effort [DOE])
Committee on Academic Freedom and Academic Tenure (AUPP), 96
communication
  about white privilege, 185–189
  listening to suggestions, 125
communities, observing, 163–164
community service, 85
competition, peers, 208–209
competitive attitudes, managing, 126
components of educator roles, 24
comrades, 69–70
confidants, 68–69
confidence-building strategies, 36–43
  adapting prior instructor's work, 41
  educational learning theories, 38–39, 40f
  guest lecturing, 41–42
  lesson plans, 40–41
  mentors, 42–43
  observing seasoned colleagues, 40
confirmation bias, 178
conflict management, 214–218
  cognitive flexibility, 214–215
  emotional regulation, 215–216
  fit of the person, 217
  self-other focus, 216
conflicts of interest, 86
connections, 51–53, 200. *See also* networking
  power connectors, 70, 202
  resilience and, 225
connectivism, 39
conscientious offloading, 87–88
consistency, 59
constituents, 69
constructivism, 38
consulting, 15
contact time, 87
contracts, 153. *See also* collaborative agreements
contributions to service, 82. *See also* time
control, patterns of, 174
coping. *See also* strategies
  collective, 200
  resistance, 201
  self-protective, 200
core competencies, 157–159
courses
  classifications, 29
  confidence-building strategies, 36–43
  evaluating teaching effectiveness, 43–46
  Fundamentals of Professional Nursing, 77
  loads, 20
COVID-19, 32, 218, 221
Cox, Tasheka, 88
CRNAs (certified registered nurse anesthetists), 154, 155
CRNPs (certified registered nurse practitioners), 152
cultural humility, 195
cultures, 103–104, 149–151

Curle, Clint, 171
curriculum, 23, 104. *See also* education
curriculum vitae, updating, 248
customer reviews, types of, 45

D

Declaration of Principles (AUPP [1915]), 96
deficiency needs, 3
degrees. *See* education; educators
dehumanization, 194
DEIB (diversity, equity, inclusion, and belonging), 112, 113, 173–175, 190–191, 194, 198–199, 218
dependability, 59
design, research, 119
determination, 231
Detweiler, Gerri, 66
Developing a Program of Research: An Essential Process for a Successful Research Career (Edwards/Roelofs), 116–117
development, contributing factors to, 115
discrimination, 182. *See also* bias; othering
Distribution of Effort (DOE), 19–22, 28, 29, 31, 33, 162
  calculating, 88–90
  entry-level positions, sample DOE, 23f
diversity, 169. *See also* othering
  decreasing quality myth, 192
  goals, 199
  in the hiring process, 197–199
  increasing, 190–193

diversity, equity, inclusion, and belonging (DEIB), 112, 113, 173–175, 190–191, 194, 198–199, 218
doctoral programs, research, 101
doctor of nursing practice (DNP), 8, 9, 29, 149–150
DOE. *See* Distribution of Effort (DOE)
double standards, 175. *See also* othering
Duckworth, Angela, 231
Dweck, Carol, 228

E

Early Career Reviewer Program (NIH), 138
education
  academic teaching, 27–29 (*see also* academic teaching)
  administration, 5–6
  clinical practice and, 141 (*see also* clinical faculty roles)
  diversity and, 170 (*see also* diversity)
  equity-minded learning, 201
  formal resilience training, 239
  research, 5
  roles of, 22–24
  scholarship, 5
  service, 4
  student interactions, 211–213
  teaching, 5
  training opportunities, 131–133
educational learning theories, 38–39, 40f
educators, 3–4

adjunct positions, 10, 146
administrative positions, 9–10
clinical-track assistant
    professors, 8–9
course loads, 20
Distribution of Effort (DOE),
    19–22 (*see also* Distribution
    of Effort [DOE])
evaluating effectiveness, 43–46
instructor positions, 9
length of appointments, 13–18
selecting positions, 10–13
special considerations of
    appointments, 18–19
tenure-track assistant
    professors, 7–8
types of entry-level
    appointments, 6–7
Edwards, Nancy, 116, 119
effectiveness, evaluating, 43–46.
    See also evaluation
    faculty feedback, 45–46
    student opinion of instructor
        (SOI) scores, 43–45, 212
    student performance, 46
effort, grit and, 231
emotional maturity, 196
emotional regulation, 215–216
emotions, negative, 224
entry-level positions, 6–7, 12*f*
    adjunct positions, 10, 146
    administrative positions, 9–10
    clinical-track assistant
        professors, 8–9
    instructor positions, 9
    sample DOE for, 23*f*
    selecting positions, 10–13
    tenure-track assistant
        professors, 7–8
    transition to, 28

environments, inclusive, 193–196
equity, 169, 198. *See also* othering
equity-minded learning, 201
eudemonic well-being, 227
evaluation
    merit evaluations, 162
    performance, 164
    productivity, 138–139
    student interactions, 211–213
exclusion, patterns of, 174
existence, purpose of, 227
expectations
    personal, 209–210
    quantity of, 22
external funding agencies, 105

F

Facebook, 65. *See also* social
    media
faculty, 7. *See also* educators
    clinical faculty roles, 141–142
        (*see also* clinical faculty roles)
    faculty member research, 103
    feedback, 45–46
    minority/foreign-born faculty,
        111–113
    othering in, 172 (*see also*
        othering)
    service at the college level,
        75–77 (*see also* service)
    shadowing, 40
    sources of stress, 206 (*see also*
        stress management)
faculty clinical practices, 155–157
Fahkry, Tony, 116
failure, 228, 229. *See also* success
fairness, institutionalizing, 182

feedback
 faculty, 45–46
 mentors and, 233
 peer review, 45–46, 130, 136, 138
 on writing, 127
fixed mindsets, 228
flexible work arrangements, 219
Floyd, George, 188
focus, 241. *See also* thriving in academia
foreign-born faculty, 111–113
formulas, strengths-based, 229
freedom, tenure and, 97
full time equivalent (FTE), 10, 18, 29, 31
Fundamentals of Professional Nursing, 77
funding
 external funding agencies, 105
 grants, 15, 121, 133–137
 intramural seed, 104–105
 using research funds, 136–137

G

Gale, Porter, 70
gender, intersectionality of race and, 175–176. *See also* othering
Gmelch, Walter, 206, 208
goals
 diversity, 199
 matching alliances with, 63–64
 mindsets and, 228
 providing to teams, 124
 for social media, 66, 67
 unrealistic personal, 209–210

graduate teaching assistants (GTAs), 28, 98, 106
grants, funding, 15, 104–105, 121, 133–137
Grantsmanship (Kraicer), 134–136
Gray, Tara, 126, 127
grit, 231
Grit (Duckworth), 231
growth mindsets, 228–229
growth needs, 3
guidelines for promotions, 162

H

Haiti Massacre, 171. *See also* othering
Hamric's Integrated Model of Advanced Practice, 158, 159*f*
Harvard University, tenure track and, 96
hierarchies
 informal, 63
 power dynamics in workplaces, 210–211
 tenure and, 11
high reliability organizations (HROs), 150–151
hiring process, diversity in, 197–199. *See also* interviews
history
 of othering, 171–172
 of tenure track, 96–98
Holocaust, 171. *See also* othering
humanism, 39
humility, cultural, 195

I

Ibitayo, Kristina, 233
implicit bias, 178
impostor syndrome, 232–233
inclusion, 169. *See also* othering
　policies and, 198
　in the workplace, 193–196
incomes. *See also* salaries
　calculating dollar value of time, 146–148
　clinical faculty roles, 144
　supplemental, 147
independent research, 115. *See also* research
individuation, 181
influencers, 63
informal hierarchies, 63
information, networking as exchange of, 53–57
insecurities, dealing with, 200–201
institutional review board (IRB), 107
instructor positions, 9
integrity, maintaining, 200–201
interactions, purpose of, 50–51
International Classification of Diseases (ICD), 218
interpersonal dynamics
　conflict management, 214–218
　stress management and, 213–218
interviews, 199, 248, 251–254. *See also* careers; hiring process
intramural seed funding, 104–105
introspection, 180–181
inventorying strengths, 54–55
IRB (institutional review board), 107

J

Jakes, T. D., 68
Jane (Journal/Author Name Estimator), 131
joining professional organizations, 83, 84–85
journals, submitting to, 131

K

King, Martin Luther, Jr., 203
Knight, Rebecca, 198
knowledge bases, building, 229
Kohll, Alan, 219
Kraicer, Jacob, 134–136

L

language, bias and, 198
Laszloffy, Tracy, 112
leadership
　lack of opportunities (othering), 173
　micromanaging team members, 126
　mindsets and, 228
　personal performance improvement plan (PIP), 139
　roles, 80, 87
　success and, 123
　teams (*see* teams)
lectures, guest lecturing, 41–42
length of appointments, 13–18
lesson plans, 40–41

licenses
    collaborative agreements and, 153
    state requirements, 151
likability, effect on hiring processes, 199
Likert scale, 44
LinkedIn, 65. *See also* social media
loyalty, 59

M

management
    conflict, 214–218
    stress (*see* stress management)
    time, 20, 21, 22
    workloads, 29–33
Mandela, Nelson, 171
manuscripts, 127. *See also* writing
Maslow's hierarchy, 3
McIntosh, Peggy, 187
meetings, scheduling, 126
memberships to professional organizations, 83, 84–85
mental health, 205. *See also* stress management
Mentoring Today's Nurses: A Global Perspective for Success (Baxley, Ibitayo, Bond), 233
mentors, 42–43, 51–53, 95, 233–238, 241
    access to, 105–107
    finding, 122, 236–238
    lack of (othering), 173
    from minority backgrounds, 202
    qualities of, 233–234
messaging, checking, 181

methods, research, 119. *See also* research
microaffirmations, 200
microaggressions, 182–186
microassaults, 183
microinsults, 183
microinvalidations, 183
micromanaging team members, 126
mindsets
    developing, 116, 126
    fixed, 228
    growth, 228–229
Mindset: The New Psychology of Success (Dweck), 228
minority/foreign-born faculty, 111–113, 173. *See also* othering
Minshew, Kathryn, 170
models, Hamric's Integrated Model of Advanced Practice, 158, 159f
motivation, 38

N

National Board of Certification and Recertification for Nurse Anesthetists (NBCRNA), 154
National Center on Complementary and Integrative Health (NCCIH), 137
National Commission to Address Racism in Nursing, 177, 196
National Institutes of Health (NIH), 108–109, 138
National League for Nursing Diversity and Inclusion Toolkit, 196

Native Americans, displacement of, 171. *See also* othering
needs
  categories of, 3
  identifying, 59–60
negative adaptation, 224
negotiations
  collaborative agreements, 154
  faculty clinical practices, 155–157
networking, 49–50
  building collaboration, 123
  definition of, 50
  as exchange of information, 53–57
  finding mentors, 122, 236–238
  interactions, 50–51
  inventorying strengths, 54–55
  purpose of, 50, 57
  resilience and, 225
  rules, 71
  social media as tool for, 64–68
  strategic classifications of, 68–71
  strategies, 57–64
  useful connections and, 51–53
Newton's Third Law of Motion, 116
Nfonoyim-Hara, Nicole Asong, 195
NIH (National Institutes of Health), 108–109, 138
normalizing burnout, 32
nurse educators, 23. *See also* educators
nurse researchers, 115–116
  building research teams, 123–126
  creating research/scholarship plans, 119–122
  defining program of research, 116–118
  developing strategic plans, 119
  evaluating productivity, 138–139
  grant funding strategies, 133–137
  as members of the scientific community, 137–138
  personal performance improvement plan (PIP), 139
  publish or perish, 126–131
  time to build teams, 125–126
  training opportunities, 131–133
nurses, shortages of, 80
nursing
  clinical, 141. (*See also* clinical faculty roles)
  curriculum, 23
  Hamric's Integrated Model of Advanced Practice, 158, 159f
  othering in, 191 (*see also* othering)
  race/racism in, 177, 178
  selecting college of nursing, 99–109

O

Obama, Michelle, 220
objectives
  mindsets and, 228
  providing to teams, 124
observing seasoned colleagues, 40
Office of Research and Development (ORED), 108
Oore, Gillin, 214, 217

opportunities
  social media and, 67 (see also social media)
  SWOT (strengths, weaknesses, opportunities, and threats) analysis, 55–57
opportunity cost, definition of, 64
organizations, service to, 81–83
othering
  in academia, 169–170, 172–175
  antidotes for in academia, 190–196
  bias, 178–182
  cultural humility, 195
  definition of, 170–171, 218
  diversity in hiring processes, 197–199
  historical perspectives on, 171–172
  inclusion in workplaces, 193–196
  intersectionality of race and gender, 175–176
  microaggressions, 182–186
  pursuing allyship, 195–196
  race/racism in nursing, 177, 178
  strategies to counter, 196–202
outputs, quality of, 22
overcommitment, 79
  calculating Distribution of Effort (DOE), 88–90
  conscientious offloading, 87–88
  risks, 86–90

P

paid service opportunities, 85–86
pandemics. See COVID-19
parent announcement (PA), 108
partnerships, 53. See also collaboration; networking
peer competition, 208–209
peer review, 45–46, 130, 136, 138
People of Color, affirmations for, 200, 202
performance
  measuring self-worth against, 209–210
  minority faculty and, 175
  stress management (see stress management)
  success and, 230 (see also success)
  teaching, 164
perseverance, 233. See also grit; resilience
personal expectations, 209–210
perspective-taking, 181
Pfeifer, Heather, 91
PhD programs, 98, 100, 101, 106, 149–150
philosophies, teaching, 37–40
physicians, collaborative agreements and, 151, 153
pilot work, funding for, 104
planning
  creating research/scholarship plans, 119–122
  developing strategic research plans, 119
  maximizing efforts, 146

personal performance improvement plan (PIP), 139
training opportunities, 131–133
using research funds, 136–137
writing grants, 133–137
platforms, 67. *See also* social media
policies, diversity in hiring processes, 197–199
positions. *See* faculty; roles; teaching; entry-level positions
Potts, Alicia, 219
power
    connectors, 70, 202
    dynamics (within workplaces), 210–211
practicality of teaching assignments, 33–34
prejudices, 171
presence, social media, 66. *See also* social media
presentations, creating research/scholarship plans, 120–121
preventing burnout, 218–221
priming, 179
productivity
    burnout and, 219
    evaluating, 138–139
    scholarly, 138–139, 207
professional contributions, 164
professional organizations
    joining, 83, 84–85
    service to, 81–83
professional service, 81. *See also* service

professors. *See also* educators
    clinical-track assistant, 8–9, 142 (*see also* clinical faculty roles)
    tenure-track assistant, 7–8
program officer (PO), 108
promotions, applying for, 164–166
publication(s)
    creating research/scholarship plans, 120
    publish or perish, 126–131
    requirements, 109–110
    writing projects in different stages, 130
Publish and Flourish: Become a Prolific Scholar (Gray), 127
purpose
    definition of, 227
    of interactions, 50–51
    of networking, 50, 57
putdowns, 182. *See also* microaggressions

Q

qualities of mentors, 233–234. *See also* mentors
quality of outputs, 22
quantity of expectations, 22

R

race, intersectionality of gender and, 175–176. *See also* othering

racial equity, 169, 173. *See also* equity; othering
racial microaffirmations, 200
racism, 188
   bias, 178–182
   microaggressions, 182–186
   in nursing, 177, 178
   strategies to counter, 196
   white privilege, 185–189
ratings, courses, 44. *See also* courses
recertification, 158. *See also* certification requirements
registered nurses (RNs), 10
relationships, 34. *See also* collaboration; networking
   choosing collaborative, 151–157
   collaboration and, 153–154
   mentors, 234, 235 (*see also* mentors)
   resilience and, 225
   rules of networking and, 71
   social media and, 64–68
   strategies, 57, 58
representation, 191
request for application (RFA), 108
research, 5, 164
   academic citizenship, 73 (*see also* academic citizenship)
   building research teams, 123–126
   clinical faculty roles, 161–164
   creating research/scholarship plans, 119–122
   culture, 103–104
   defining program of, 116–118
   design, 119
   determining impact of, 116
   developing strategic plans, 119
   evaluating productivity, 138–139
   faculty member, 103
   finding mentors, 122
   institutional research expectations, 99–101
   nurse researchers, 115–116 (*see also* nurse researchers)
   personal performance improvement plan (PIP), 139
   publish or perish, 126–131
   selecting areas of, 162–163
   submitting to journals, 131
   support, 101–103
   support from dean of, 107–109
   tenure-track assistant professors, 7–8
   time to build teams, 125–126
   training opportunities, 131–133
   types of customer reviews, 45
   using research funds, 136–137
research-intensive institution (R01), 162
resilience, 224–231
   definition of, 224
   formal resilience training, 239
   growth mindsets and, 228–229
   strengths-based psychology, 229–230
resistance coping, 201
resources, othering and, 176
resumes, 199, 248. *See also* careers; hiring process
reviews, minority faculty, 175
risks, overcommitment, 86–90
RNs (registered nurses), 10
Robinett, Judy, 70, 71
Rockquemore, Kerry Ann, 112

Roelofs, Susan, 116, 119
roles
  academic, 7–8 (*see also* educators)
  academic citizenship, 73–74 (*see also* academic citizenship; service)
  assigning based on expertise, 124, 125
  clinical faculty, 141–142 (*see also* clinical faculty roles)
  education, 22–24
  leadership, 80, 87
  service, 77 (*see also* service)
rules, networking and, 71
Rwandan Genocide, 171. *See also* othering

S

salaries
  9-month appointments, 16–18
  clinical faculty roles, 144
scheduling
  increasing writing productivity, 127, 128–129
  team meetings, 126
Scholarly Affairs Committee, 76
scholarly productivity, 7–8, 138–139, 207
scholarship, 5, 164
  clinical faculty roles, 161–164
  creating research/scholarship plans, 119–122
  culture, 103–104
  incorporating in teaching, 129
  productivity, 99
  selecting areas of, 162–163
  tenure track and, 101
science, evaluating, 116
scientists, 115–116, 137–138
scores, Student Opinion of Instructor (SOI), 43–45, 212
searching for mentors, 42–43
security, tenure and, 97
selecting positions, 10–13
self-actualization, 3, 157, 227
self-care, 87, 88, 206. *See also* stress management
self-efficacy, 33
self-other focus, 216
self-protective coping, 200
service, 4, 73–74. *See also* academic citizenship
  calculating Distribution of Effort (DOE), 88–90
  at the college level, 75–77
  commitment contact hours, 89*t*–90*t*
  community, 85
  conscientious offloading, 87–88
  definition of, 73
  joining professional organizations, 83, 84–85
  opportunities for, 74, 75, 78, 79, 82, 83, 86
  paid/unpaid opportunities, 85–86
  to professional organizations, 81–83
  risk of overcommitment, 86–90
  time commitments to, 81, 82
  types of opportunities, 90–91
  to the university, 78–80
Set Boundaries, Find Peace: A Guide to Reclaiming Yourself (Tawwab), 215

sexual and gender minorities (SGMs), 175, 176. *See also* othering
shadowing faculty, 40
skills, acquiring new, 228–229. *See also* mindsets; resilience
slowing down, 181
social media as tool for networking, 64–68
SOI (Student Opinion of Instructor) scores, 43–45, 212
solutions, offering, 60
sources of stress in academia, 206–213
    peer competition, 208–209
    power dynamics (within workplaces), 210–211
    student interactions, 211–213
    teaching assignment overload, 207
    unrealistic personal expectations, 209–210
Southern Nursing Research Society (SNRS), 228
specialty considerations, 159–161
startup funds, availability of, 133. *See also* funding
Statement of Principles of Academic Freedom and Tenure (1940), 97
state requirements
    collaboration and, 159, 160
    licenses, 151
strategies
    to address microaggressions, 184
    building resilience, 224–228
    to combat implicit bias, 180–182
    confidence-building, 36–43
    to counter othering, 199–202
    to counter racism, 196
    cultural humility, 195
    to deal with imposter syndrome, 232–233
    developing strategic research plans, 119
    diversity in hiring processes, 197–199
    educational learning theories, 38–39, 40*f*
    for failure, 228, 229
    grant funding, 133–137
    inclusion in workplaces, 193–196
    increasing diversity, 190–193
    interviews, 252–254
    networking, 57–64
    personal performance improvement plan (PIP), 139
    publish or perish, 126–131
    pursuing allyship, 195–196
    submitting to journals, 131
    for success, 115–116
    team building, 125
    writing projects in different stages, 130
strengths
    definition of strength, 229
    inventorying, 54–55
    sharing, 60–61
    SWOT (strengths, weaknesses, opportunities, and threats) analysis, 55–57
strengths-based psychology, 229–230
stress management, 205–206
    adapting to stress, 224 (*see also* resilience)
    conflict management, 214–218

interpersonal dynamics and, 213–218
peer competition, 208–209
power dynamics (within workplaces), 210–211
sources of stress in academia, 206–213
student interactions, 211–213
teaching assignment overload, 207
unrealistic personal expectations, 209–210
work-life balance (preventing burnout), 218–221
student interactions, 211–213
Student Life Committee, 76
Student Opinion of Instructor (SOI) scores, 43–45, 212
student performance, 46
submitting to journals, 131
success
    in academia, 223–224 (*see also* thriving in academia)
    contributing factors to, 115
    defining program of research, 116–118
    in interviews, 254
    leadership capabilities and, 123
    performance and, 230
    training opportunities, 131–133
supplemental incomes, 147. *See also* incomes
support, 200
    from dean of research, 107–109
    othering and, 176, 191
    tenure track, 101–103
surveys, 43–45
SWOT (strengths, weaknesses, opportunities, and threats) analysis, 55–57, 101

T

take two concept, 182
talent, 229. *See also* skills
Tawwab, Nedra Glover, 215
teaching, 5. *See also* education; educators
    academic citizenship, 73 (*see also* academic citizenship)
    academic teaching, 27–29 (*see also* academic teaching)
    assignment overload, 207 (*see also* stress management)
    calculating workloads, 31t
    clinical faculty roles, 141–149 (*see also* clinical faculty roles)
    confidence-building strategies, 36–43
    evaluating effectiveness, 43–46
    incomes, 146 (*see also* incomes)
    incorporating scholarship, 129
    load practicality, 33t
    managing workloads, 29–33
    performance, 164
    philosophies, 37–40
    practicality of teaching assignments, 33–34
teams
    assigning roles based on expertise, 124
    building research, 123–126
    micromanaging team members, 126
    providing goals and objectives, 124
    scheduling team meetings, 126

stages of building, 125–126
writing, 130
tenure
    definition of, 97
    Distribution of Effort (DOE), 21
    hierarchies and, 11
    minority/foreign-born faculty, 111–113
tenure track. *See also* colleges
    access to mentors, 105–107
    culture, 103–104
    faculty member research, 103
    falling behind, 109–111
    history of, 96–98
    institutional research expectations, 99–101
    intramural seed funding, 104–105
    publication requirements, 109–110
    selecting college of nursing, 99–109
    struggling with teaching and research, 110–111
    support, 101–103
    support from dean of research, 107–109
tenure-track assistant professors, 7–8
theories, educational learning, 38–39, 40*f*
threats, 55–57, 224
thriving in academia, 223–224
    definition of thrive, 193, 223, 224
    formal resilience training, 239
    grit, 231
    imposter syndrome, 232–233

mentors, 233–338
resilience, 224–231 (*see also* resilience)
wisdom and advice, 240–249
time
    to build teams, 125–126
    calculating dollar value of, 146–148
    commitments to service, 81, 82 (*see also* service)
    conscientious offloading, 87–88
    contact time, 87
    management, 20, 21, 22
    practicality of teaching assignments, 33–34
    teaching assignment overload, 35–36
    workload management, 29–33
Tochluk, Shelly, 187, 188
tokenism, 194
tools, social media, 64–68. *See also* strategies
tragedy, adapting to, 224
training opportunities, 131–133, 239. *See also* education
transatlantic slave trade, 171. *See also* othering
transitions, 10–13
trauma, adapting to, 224
traveling, distance to work, 148–149
Truong, Kimberly, 191
trust, building, 57–59
Tuckman, Bruce, 125
Twitter, 65. *See also* social media
Type A personalities, 209

U–V

United Kingdom (UK), racial equity in, 173
university. *See also* college
service to, 78–80
University of Michigan Center for Research on Learning and Teaching, 39
University of Minnesota Center for Education and Innovation, 39
unpaid service opportunities, 85–86
usefulness, definition of, 51
U.S. Preventive Medicine, 228

value
adding to networks, 70
attribution, 179
Veterans Affairs Medical Center (VAMC), 106

W

weaknesses
acknowledging, 62
focusing on, 230
SWOT (strengths, weaknesses, opportunities, and threats) analysis, 55–57
well-being, eudemonic, 227
white faculty, 174. *See also* faculty; othering
white privilege, 185–189. *See also* microaggressions; othering
communication about, 188
definition of, 186, 187
Witnessing Whiteness (Tochluk), 187
work-life balance, 218–221
workloads
calculating, $31t$
clinical faculty roles, 142, 144, 147
Distribution of Effort (DOE), 33 (*see also* Distribution of Effort [DOE])
incomes (*see* incomes)
practicality of teaching assignments, 33–34
teaching assignment overload, 35–36
workplaces
conflict resolution and, 217–218
flexible work arrangements, 219
inclusion in, 193–196
power dynamics within, 210–211
World Health Organization (WHO), 218
writing
changing focus of, 129–130
grants, 133–137
increasing productivity, 127, 128–129
peer review, 130, 136
projects in different stages, 130
publish or perish, 126–131
submitting to journals, 131
teams, 130

Y–Z

Your Network Is Your Net Worth
(Gale), 70

Ziglar, Zig, 239

www.ingramcontent.com/pod-product-compliance
Lightning Source LLC
Chambersburg PA
CBHW052057300426
44117CB00013B/2169